OPHTHALMOLOGY

THE ESSENTIALS

David Miller, MD

Associate Professor of Ophthalmology
Harvard Medical School
Chief of Ophthalmology
Beth Israel Hospital, Boston

Houghton Mifflin Professional Publishers
Medical Division
Boston

Library of Congress Cataloging in Publication Data

Miller, David, 1931–
  Ophthalmology, the essentials.

  Includes bibliographical references and index.
  1. Eye—Diseases and defects.   2. Ophthalmology.
I. Title.   DNLM: 1. Eye diseases.   WW100.3 M647o
RE46.M54   617.7   79-9828
ISBN 0-89289-325-7

Any editorial inquiries should be directed to
Morton K. Rubinstein, MD, Editorial Director.

ISBN   0-89289-325-7

LCCCN   79-9828

Cover design by Margaret Ong Tsao.

Foreword

It is clear that Dr. Miller's *Ophthalmology: The Essentials* is not just another medical textbook, for it distinguishes itself from the available ophthalmologic texts in two important ways: it is appropriately concise and selective in its approach, and it is written in a lucid, narrative style. Its style, in fact, may suit some readers better than others, but it certainly demonstrates that a medical book need not be dull and unnecessarily formidable. The student will find Dr. Miller's approach of considerable value, because it places the specialty of ophthalmology in proper perspective for the nonspecialist.

Unlike other textbooks of ophthalmology, *Ophthalmology: The Essentials* was written specifically for the medical student who must rotate in rapid succession through the medical and surgical subspecialties. With this limitation in mind, Dr. Miller has produced a book that clearly distinguishes the common from the exotic and the essential from the unessential. It emphasizes the eye conditions, emergencies, and procedures that every student should take from the medical school course in ophthalmology, and that every physician should know, regardless of his specialty. In addition to its succinct discussions of ocular anatomy, diagnosis, and treatment, this book provides the reader with a sound understanding of the pathophysiology of the major disease processes, each of which is treated in appropriate detail. Dr. Miller's chapters on ocular emergencies and medical treatment of eye conditions will prove of great practical value to both the student and the practitioner.

Medical students are not the only group who will benefit from this new approach to medical textbooks. Optometrists, nurses, and other health personnel who must deal with eye problems will also find this book invaluable. Its storehouse of information, concision, and readability make *Ophthalmology: The Essentials* unique—and that in itself is a remarkable accomplishment for a medical textbook.

Claes H. Dohlman, MD
Professor and Chairman
Department of Ophthalmology
Harvard Medical School

Preface

Yesterday, four medical journals and a glossy product brochure arrived in the mail. Today, the postman delivered the surgical text I ordered last month, along with two medical newsletters and an FDA drug bulletin. This amount of mail far surpasses my reading time and ability, and constantly reminds me that the entries into the world brain are doubling every seven years. This should come as no surprise; half of all the scientists ever born are alive today (and, obviously, publishing). Remarkable, certainly, and perhaps even laudable—but pity the poor student who is asked to absorb, assimilate, interpret, and utilize this ever-rising mountain of facts. What is he to do?

The problem resembles the one faced by the creative scientist, who must spot the promising clue amid the daily output of discussions, data, and details. The novelist Pearl Buck felt that "the truly creative mind, in any field, is no more than this: a human creature born abnormally, inhumanly sensitive. To him, a touch is a blow, a sound is a noise, a misfortune is a tragedy, and a joy an ecstasy." If we can transfer this lesson to the problems of education, we see that the truly creative scientist must cultivate the ability to distinguish essential from unessential information. But if you are not yet able to do this, how do you handle all of this information?

In evaluating those millions of income tax returns, the Internal Revenue Service has developed a system of flagging the most common sources of cheating within selected groups. Distilling statistically significant material is the key. This book uses a similar technique. For example, it is true that there are over 50 known causes of a red, painful eye, but a knowledge of only five common causes will allow the physician to deal effectively with 95% of all the red eyes seen in an emergency room; and so only these five causes are discussed in the chapter on eye emergencies.

Most authors of texts for medical students recognize that the author's role is to emphasize the common and to gloss the exotic. The adage "When you hear hoofbeats think of horses, not zebras," reminds us of this necessity. But the author addresses not only students, but also his peers, who function as critics for publishing companies and journals and who are concerned with depth of knowledge, completeness of coverage, and professional dignity. I hope that these critics are similarly concerned with the needs of the undergraduate medical student, for this book was conceived and written to help the physician-in-training develop a foundation for understanding ophthalmology. It is also my hope that various other people—including optometrists and graduate nurses—will find this book of value.

The book would not have been possible without the help and advice of many people. I owe deep thanks to Dr. Edward Ryan for writing the original drafts of the retina chapter, and to Ms. Ann Ripley for her draft of the chapter on eye myths. Special thanks go to Dr. Peter Gudas for his guidance on the chapter on pharmacology, to Dr. Howard Feldman for his help on the systemic disease chapter, to Dr. David Campbell for his work on the glaucoma chapter, to Dr. George Powers for his painstaking review of the manuscript as seen through the eyes of a medical student, and to all the Harvard Medical School students who offered constructive criticism and encouragement. Finally, many thanks to Mrs. Brina Hurwitz and Mrs. Sheila Schott for those many hours of manuscript typing and retyping.

David Miller, MD
Boston, Massachusetts
January 1979

Introduction

It all began about 300 million years ago when the "Evolutionary Council" started research and development on "Project Oculus." The first step was merely a small light-sensitive spot on the back of a one-celled animal. Through time, each component of the eye underwent many changes before the mammalian eye evolved. It may interest some to see how nature experimented with the eyes of lower species:

1. Most fish have no eyelids.

2. Snakes have translucent lids that protect their eyes as they burrow, while allowing them to see large objects.

3. Birds have a third translucent lid that can be closed without interfering with vision but that does not sparkle, thus helping to camouflage them from predators.

4. The snake changes the focus of its lens by back-and-forth movement, whereas the lens of a mammal's eye changes shape.

5. The nautilus, a mollusk related to the squid, has no lens at all, but simply a tiny opening at the front of its eye that causes its eye to function in a manner similar to that of a pinhole camera.

6. Copilia, a pinhead-sized copepod, has but one light-sensitive retinal cell, which is attached to a thin muscle. As copilia's corneal lens creates an image, the muscle moves the retinal cell back and forth. This system can scan the image at the focal plane at rates up to five times a second.*

---

*Mueller CG, Rudolph M: *Light and Vision.* New York, Time-Life Books, 1966, pp 16–30.

The motto of evolution must indeed be an eye for every need. In the first chapter we will describe in some detail the eye of man and its unique characteristics.

Evolution has fashioned eyes that not only satisfy the visual needs of man, but that also repair themselves. Nicks and scratches of the highly polished corneal surface are filled in first by migrating epithelial cells. The surface is then refinished perfectly by rapidly dividing epithelial cells. In the event of a small puncture or laceration of the cornea, the iris functions as an instant repair kit, swelling with fluid and ballooning forward to plug the corneal wound. And when a sudden rush of wind swirls dirt or dust into our eyes, waterfalls of tears almost instantly wash away the annoying particles.

Our eyes not only repair superficial injury, but also seem to resist certain forms of generalized disease. The cornea, with the exception of the transitional limbal zone, never develops cancer. Nor does the lens. The vascularized components of the eye—the iris, choroid, and retina—are subject to cancer, but the incidence of malignant changes are exceedingly low when compared to cancers of the lung, breast, or colon.

With such a vigorous repair and maintenance program operating in the eye, one might legitimately wonder why there is need for eye doctors. But evolution seems to have neglected the problem of aging. The eye of a middle-aged man, for example, loses the power of accommodation, and must be helped with reading glasses. Senile cataracts must be removed surgically. Glaucoma becomes a problem after 40 and must be treated. Each of these problems is described in a different chapter of this book.

Second, evolution has not had time to respond to the changes of modern civilization. As we advance, society's blind do not perish, but they are protected; they enjoy full lives and have children. Because many blinding diseases are passed along genetically, we must contend with diabetic retinopathy, retinitis pigmentosa, and retinal detachments, to name but a few. These problems are all considered in the chapters on retinal disease and ocular manifestations of systemic disease.

As we come full circle, we begin to appreciate the magnificence of ocular evolution while still appreciating the need to diagnose and treat a sizable number of ocular problems not addressed by evolution. It is my hope that this book will fill in the details of the circle.

Chapter 1

Structure and Function of the Eye

In G.K. Chesterton's story "The Invisible Man," a postman enters a building, commits a murder, and walks away unnoticed. Although the man is entirely visible, his presence is so routine that it fails to trigger the attention of those in the building. Thus, as Chesterton illustrated, vision is more than the mere registration of a retinal image; it is also a processing of such images by the brain. The million ganglion cells of the retina transmit 500 electrical signals along the optic nerve each second (in computer language, the equivalent of one-half billion bits of information per second[1]), and the brain is constantly sorting this stream of information, selecting only those visual events that are new or important and correlating apparently random images with past visual experience.

The Role of the Brain

The brain cannot interpret everything it sees from birth. As the child develops, it catalogues visual experiences much as one stores color slides in a memory book. What the retina registers is then always compared to our cerebral slide collection, and what we finally think we see is a perception of the slide and not the actual scene.

Though awesome and complex, this interpretive process of the brain is not foolproof, sometimes mistaking appearances for reality. For example, the moon on the horizon appears to be an enormous object. Yet how large is it really? We know that it subtends an angle of only $1/2$ degree. If the circular dome of the heavens is 180°, the moon is 1/360 of the circle, or 1/100,000 part of the entire heavenly dome, and can be blocked from view by holding a quarter in front of the eye. But the brain expects the

1

moon to be large on the horizon, and so it interprets it to be larger than the actual retinal image.[2]

Very little is known about how the brain processes images, although this problem has long been a subject of scientific interest. Two Harvard researchers have taken some first steps in elucidating the process in cats and monkeys.[3] They showed that only certain cells in the visual cortex were excited when the animal looked at a horizontal bar, while other brain cells fired when the bar was tipped obliquely. Finally, different sets of brain cells responded to target movement in one direction only. From this and other work we are beginning to understand how the brain-retina complex extracts certain basic elements of each scene and transmits this information to special cells in the brain, which then reconstitutes a mental impression of that specific scene.

Occasionally, nature itself works very informative experiments. In one such instance, an eight-month-old boy lost his sight as a result of a corneal infection in both eyes, which left his corneas dense, white, and scarred.[4] He accumulated no further visual experience until age 34, when an artificial cornea was surgically implanted. After the operation this patient had difficulty separating important objects from meaningless backgrounds—differentiating a tie from a shirt, for example. He learned to do only a few things with his new vision, such as seeing the food on his plate, avoiding large objects, reading large signs, and recognizing certain colors. The patient described his situation as follows: "I had never had the experience of seeing. Only with great effort was I able to see the outline of a person or of obstacles against the light. I used to have some idea of space in mind. I never had a clear idea about the distance of objects from me. When I returned home I began to walk around alone. I can see people, although I cannot understand their faces."

Such patients are not fooled by optical illusions because their visual memory is insufficient to influence their retinal imagery. Unfortunately, most patients who regain sight after being blind during their formative period can never exploit the visual world as sighted people are able to do. (This condition, called *amblyopia,* is discussed in Chapter 10.) They often become severely depressed when their sight is restored, perhaps from frustration.

As these animal and human experiments illustrate, the student of ophthalmology not only must learn the anatomy and function of the eye, but also must know the relevant brain pathways concerned with sight.

The Anatomy and Function of the Eye

Figure 1-1 is a diagram of the eye. Although only an inch in diameter, it is crammed with almost every type of tissue found in the rest of the body,

ANATOMY OF THE EYE

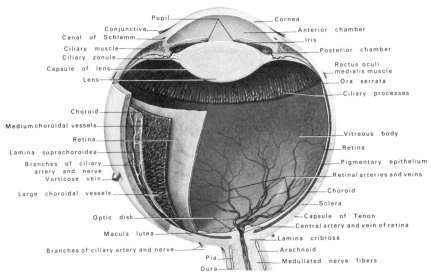

Figure 1-1. Anatomy of the eye. (Courtesy of Lederle Laboratories, Inc.)

along with a few unique varieties. Let us now look at each element of the eye in more detail.

Cornea

The cornea and lens of the eye are the two key optical elements responsible for sharp retinal imagery. Their optics are similar to those of an advanced lens design, and yet they are living structures. The cornea, for example, repairs many of its own nicks and scratches.

The *cornea,* the tough, front covering of the eye, serves as its most powerful focusing element, being about three times as powerful as the lens. The secret of the cornea's optical effectiveness consists in its shape and composition (Fig. 1-2). It has a steep, spherical shape centrally, and tends to flatten peripherally, thus eliminating *spherical aberration,* a distortion seen in all man-made, single-element spherical lenses. The cornea is made of strong, transparent collagen fibers that are embedded in a ground substance. The refractive index (light-bending power) of the cornea is very similar to that of water. Thus, the cornea refracts light rays well when surrounded by air, but its effectiveness is almost completely neutralized under water. Even in fish, the optic power of the cornea is neutralized by water; and so the fish eye focuses almost exclusively by a very powerful lens.

In humans, the corneal surface is smooth, like any effective optical surface. Its five rows of epithelial cells continually repair any nicks or cracks that develop, and the thin film of tears over the cornea washes the

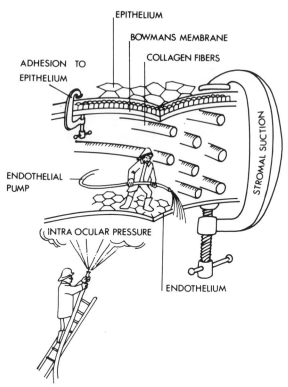

Figure 1-2. Close-up of the corneal microstructure, showing the epithelium, endothelium, and intervening stromal fibers, and the forces that keep the cornea clear and compact. (Artists: David Lobel and Laurel Cook.)

surface smooth each time the lid blinks. A dense network of nerves stimulates blinking and tearing, thus preventing wind-blown particles from becoming embedded in the corneal surface. Nevertheless, some situations can overwhelm the eye's ability to protect itself. For example, racehorses running in a close pack on a cinder track are very susceptible to corneal scratches from particulate matter blown up into their eyes. Some are now fitted with soft clear contact lenses to protect their corneas. A more detailed description of the cornea appears in the chapter on corneal disease.

Lens

The *lens* is made of densely packed, elongated, nonnucleated, transparent cells (Fig. 1-3). Throughout life, new layers of these cells are added, much as a tree accumulates rings as it grows. With the use of a slit lamp (discussed more fully in Chapter 2), experts can actually estimate a patient's age by counting these layers.[5]

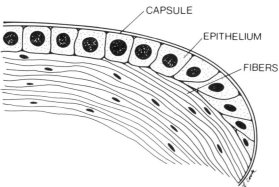

Figure 1-3. Anatomy of the eye-lens microstructure. (Artist: Laurel Cook.)

The focusing power of the lens, as of the cornea and all artificial lenses, depends on its index of refraction and shape. The mammalian lens is set apart from artificial lenses by its ability to accommodate, i.e., to change its focus by changing its shape. The transparent cells that make up the lens are elastic, and the entire lens is wrapped in a very thin and highly elastic capsule. The lens would assume a spherical shape (Fig. 1-4) if it were not for the few hundred *zonules,* or fine ligaments, that are inserted around the edge of the lens and that pull it into a flatter shape. The zonules, in turn, are attached to the ciliary body, which contains the ring-shaped *ciliary muscle.* When the ciliary muscle contracts, it moves forward and the circle of muscle becomes smaller. Both actions allow the zonules to slacken and the lens to bulge. The amount of ciliary muscle contraction and subsequent accommodative focusing is controlled by the clarity of the retinal image as interpreted by the brain and is thus, in the final analysis, controlled by the brain.[6]

Amplitude of accommodation may be said to be measured in *diopters* (D), an optical unit obtained by dividing by 100 the closest distance in centimeters that a small object can be focused clearly (explained more fully in Chapter 5). The accommodative amplitude of a child is about 15 D, i.e., the child can keep a fly in focus as it moves from the far side of the room to within 5 ½ cm of his eyes. Although the power of the cornea is neutralized under water, a 10-year-old can read newspaper print under water on a bright, sunny day because his accommodative power, plus the pinhole effect of his constricted pupil, compensate for this neutralization. (The pinhole effect is discussed in Chapter 5.) Unhappily, this range of accommodation decreases with age as the lens capsule thickens and stiffens and as the internal lens fibers become more densely packed, losing elasticity. The ciliary muscle hypertrophies in an attempt to compensate for increased lens stiffness, but to no avail. By age 45, the accommodative power may be down to 3 D; by age 65, the ability to accommodate is usually gone, and reading glasses become a necessity (Table 1-1).

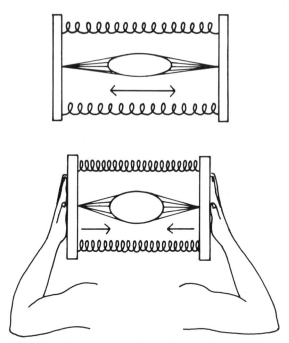

Figure 1-4. Mechanism of accommodation. The hands represent the contracting ciliary muscle that slackens the zonules, allowing the lens to bulge. (Artists: David Lobel and Laurel Cook.)

Another age-related change in the lens is yellowing, which tends to filter out bluish colors. Many older artists tend to use deeper blues, for instance, so that they themselves can see the color, and after having a cataract removed some patients happily report that they can once more see the deeper and more intense blues.

When the lens is injured or affected by systemic disease or local inflammation, it develops opacities called *cataracts*. The severity of a cataract is defined by the degree of opacity—the more opaque, the more severe the cataract. Cataracts are the subject of Chapter 8.

Iris

Iris is Greek for rainbow, and irises are seen in a variety of colors and shades. Most caucasian babies have blue irises during the first year of life. The blue color is not produced by pigment, but from the Rayleigh light-scattering produced by the fine collagen fibers of the iris. In time, melanin pigment will be placed in the body of the iris, producing the various adult colors. An albino patient has no iris pigment, and so the many blood vessels of the iris, plus the light-scattering effect, give it a translucent gray-pink appearance. Iris pigmentation is indirectly linked to

Table 1-1. Accommodative Power as a Function of Age

Age (years)	Near-Point (cm)	Amplitude of Accommodation (D)
10	7	14
15	8	12
20	10	10
25	12	8.5
30	14	7
35	18	5.5
40	22	4.5
45	28	3.5
50	40	2.5
55	51	1.75
60	100	1
65	200	0.50
70	400	0.25

the sympathetic nervous system, and so a young patient sustaining trauma to the sympathetic chain on one side of the neck will have a lighter colored iris on that side. Also, patients with brown or hazel eyes have a more sensitive oculocardiac reflex (a slowing of the heart when the eye is pressed or when traction is placed on the medial rectus muscle) than those with blue or gray eyes.[7]

Microscopically, the iris is about as thick as the fabric of a cotton dress (0.25 mm) and balloonlike in nature. This quality allows it to fall forward spontaneously and plug up penetrating corneal lacerations, a maneuver that keeps the aqueous from running out of the eye and, thus, that maintains the integrity of the eye until healing has occurred.

Surrounding the pupil is a small collar of muscle known as the *sphincter.* Located more peripherally are the dilating muscle fibers that pull the pupil open (Fig. 1-5). The body of the iris, known as the *stroma,* has those extra pigment cells that give the iris its distinctive color. Finally, every iris (except that in the albinotic individual) is backed by a heavy black pigment layer that prevents oncoming light from striking the retina except through the pupil.[8]

Some irises look odd because ophthalmologists have surgically altered their shape in operations for cataract or glaucoma. Figure 1-6 shows the different types of iridectomies.

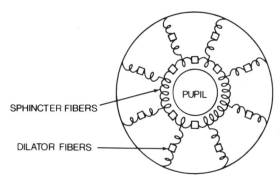

Figure 1-5. Diagrammatic representation of the iris musculature.

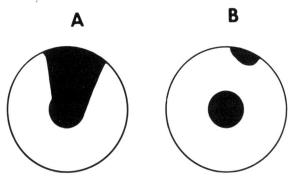

Figure 1-6. Types of iridectomies. **A** Basal. **B** Peripheral.

Pupil

The pupil functions just as the f-stop* on the camera, i.e., to help control light striking the retina. Anyone familiar with cameras knows that even an expensive camera with a wide range of f-stops cannot take pictures under all lighting conditions with only one type of film. The eye works in the same way. The pupil can dilate to a diameter of 8 mm and constrict to about 2 mm, thus yielding a range of pupil area of 16 to 1. Yet the eye can see over a range of about a million light units. Therefore, the human pupil can make only a small contribution toward the maintenance of constant retinal illumination.

Researchers in Cambridge, England discovered that an eye with a normally sized pupil has an absolute light threshold (i.e., minimum amount of light detectable) one-tenth that of a control eye with an enlarged pupil during the first few minutes of dark adaptation.[9] Could

---

*There is a numbered wheel on most cameras. Each number describes the lighting conditions under which a properly exposed picture can be taken. The numbers are called f-stops. Thus, if the camera is set at f-18 or f-11, the "pupil" is small and set to take a picture in bright light. On the other hand, a setting of f-2 allows one to take a picture in dim light.

this fact have any real significance? Looking down the evolutionary scale, we note that the cat's pupil can range from a 12.5-mm diameter circle to a slit 0.2 mm in width or an area range of 135 times, which is almost 10 times greater than the human range. For a moment, let us picture a catlike animal being pursued in bright sunlight. Suddenly, it leaps into the apparent safety of a dark cave. A change in pupillary area of 135 times may be very significant in achieving a rapid and useful dark adaptation helpful for survival.

As it does in response to bright light, the pupil also constricts and creates a pinhole effect when an object is held close to the eye. This effect, as explained in Figure 1-7, helps to sharpen the focus of anything we see. In ordinary indoor lighting the pupil is 3–6 mm in diameter, and it gets a bit smaller with age. Most of us have pupils of similar size in both eyes, but about 10% of the normal population has a slight size asymmetry known as *anisocoria*. A large anisocoria often indicates brain disease or injury and should be evaluated by a neurologist. Very small pupils sometimes suggest heroin or morphine addiction, or in patients over 40 small pupils may suggest that they have glaucoma and are taking pilocarpine eyedrops, which constrict the pupil.

The pupil, if observed under high magnification, is in constant motion. One of the reasons proposed is that control of its size is based on an intricate feedback system.[10] In electronics, self-tuning or self-focusing controls usually have a slight jitter or static unless extremely elaborate compensatory circuits are used. Thus the microscopic movement of the pupil (known as *hippus*), which is virtually unnoticeable and would have required an enormous amount of extra neurologic circuitry to eliminate, is an example of nature's economy.

Finally, the pupil can be exploited as an easily observed indicator of brain activity. One of the criteria used to determine whether brain death has occurred in a drowning or cardiac arrhythmia patient is pupil size and reaction to a flashlight. In brain death, the pupil dilates to about 6 mm and does not constrict when light is shown on the eye. And psychologists have discovered that the pupil is also an objective indicator of the emotional state: presenting the picture of a nude woman to a male subject, for instance, will likely cause his pupils to dilate.[11] The advertising industry also has made use of pupillography in determining how to attract the attention of the average consumer faced with hundreds of different advertisements in the course of a week. To test the effectiveness of ads, advertising agencies may present a series of ads to a group of subjects, following the pupillographic responses and selecting the ad that causes pupillary dilation.

Anterior Chamber and the Aqueous Humor

Located between the iris and the cornea is a fluid-filled space, the *anterior chamber*. It roughly resembles a triangle on cross section (Fig. 1-8), with

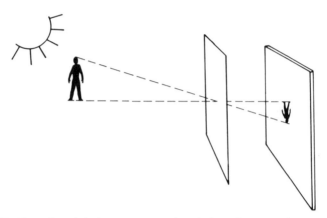

Figure 1-7. How the pinhole camera works. Only a few rays from a specified region of the target are allowed to reach a single region of the screen through the hole. All other rays from the region are blocked. Thus, an inverted image is constructed only from those rays penetrating the hole. (Artist: David Lobel.)

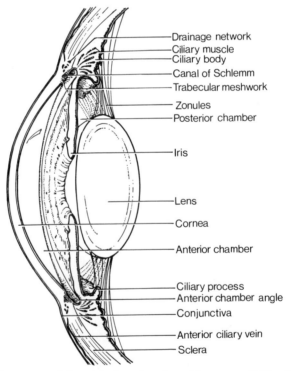

Drainage network
Ciliary muscle
Ciliary body
Canal of Schlemm
Trabecular meshwork

Zonules
Posterior chamber

Iris

Lens

Cornea

Anterior chamber

Ciliary process
Anterior chamber angle
Conjunctiva

Anterior ciliary vein
Sclera

Figure 1-8. Anatomy of the anterior chamber. (Courtesy of Merck, Sharpe & Dohme.)

the apex at the corneal center and the other two angles formed between the iris and the peripheral cornea. The anterior chamber is filled with a clear fluid, the *aqueous humor*, or, simply, aqueous. Secreted by the ciliary body, aqueous nourishes and bathes the cornea and lens, both of which must remain transparent and free of blood vessels. Therefore, the aqueous is similar to blood in composition, but is clear because it is acellular and has a lower protein content.

The aqueous is produced by the epithelial cells of the ciliary body (see next section). These cells extract important components from blood passing through nearby vessels and discharge these components into the anterior chamber. The fresh aqueous flows over the lens and the corneal endothelium and leaves through the filtration structures located at the angles of the triangular chamber. If these angles or the small pores within them are blocked, aqueous cannot exit easily, and the pressure within the eye rises, causing a condition known as glaucoma. Glaucoma is the subject of Chapter 9.

Aqueous that is not crystal-clear indicates that disease may be present or that trauma has occurred. If the eye sustains a blow, for example, a shock wave is created in the aqueous. This shock wave can avulse blood vessels located at the margins of the iris and result in bleeding into the anterior chamber. This condition is known as *hyphema*. If the angles become blocked by cells or acellular debris, the intraocular pressure may rise to dangerous levels. Fortunately, in most cases fixed macrophages lining the pores of the filtering angle are able to phagocytize the accumulated cells and debris, and proper flow of aqueous is reestablished within a week.

Ciliary Body

The *ciliary body* lies between the iris and the *choroid* (see next section). Four functions can legitimately be assigned to this structure. First, its sphincter-type muscle controls the focus of the eye lens (known as accommodation) and thus continually keeps a crisp image on the retina.[12] Second, its epithelial cells are the anchoring posts for the lens zonules. Third, it is the ciliary epithelium that secretes the aqueous humor.

Finally, because the ciliary muscle is attached to the filtering meshwork, contraction of the muscle can pull these pores open and thus improve drainage. For example, pilocarpine eyedrops (used to treat glaucoma) are known to cause the ciliary muscle to contract. These eyedrops improve aqueous outflow by activating the ciliary muscle pulling on the pores of the filtration angle.

Anterior uveitis is an inflammation of the ciliary body that results in a discharge of pus into the anterior chamber. This exudate is viscous and is capable of blocking the filtering angles and gluing the iris to the lens or cornea. (See Chapter 12 for a more complete discussion.)

Choroid

The *choroid* is the backward extension of the iris and the ciliary body. It is sandwiched between the *sclera* on the outside and a connective tissue sheet called *Bruch's membrane* on the inside. Highly vascular, it consists of a complex four-layer network of blood vessels. This network serves to supply the enormous nutritional requirements of the *retina*, which is extremely active metabolically. The retina also gains a good deal of heat from the light that strikes it. This heat is dissipated by the constant flow of blood through the choroid.

Pigment cells are interspersed among the vessels of the network. Melanin, the choroid's dark-brown pigment, captures stray light, reducing internal reflections, and prevents outside light from leaking in through the sclera. On rare occasions, the melanin cells of the choroid transform and produce a malignancy known as choroidal melanoma. If the malignancy goes undetected and grows large, enucleation (removal of an eye) is often required.

The major function of the choroid is to provide nutrition and cooling to the overlying retina (see Fig. 1-9). The choroidal arterial supply[13] is segmental, with no anastomoses between adjacent arteries. Surprisingly, occlusion of any of the entering posterior ciliary arteries does not result in a choroidal infarct. Such protection lies in the arrangement of the choroidal veins which overlap adjacent areas. Thus, in the event of an occlusion of a short posterior ciliary artery, blood from an open artery fills a corresponding vein. This vein drains into a bigger vein which originally drained the occluded segment. Now, blood from this last vein will flow backward into the occluded segment and supply the needed blood in the reverse direction. Although the vein cannot pump blood forward, it is helped by the pumping of the intraocular pulsation. Thus, arterial segments communicate through choroidal veins, which incidentally have an oxygen content very similar to that of choroidal arteries.

Retina

The surface area of the *retina* is about 17 cm^2, its thickness is about 0.2 mm, and it looks rather unimposing, just a clear membrane with some fine red lines running through it.

The retina contains the eye's light-sensitive receptor cells, and functions in a manner analogous to that of a TV camera, which can record images focused on it, process those images instantaneously, and respond automatically to changes in light levels via a sensing system that regulates the size of the iris diaphragm. The retina can do all this and more.

Retinal sensitivity covers a range of 10,000,000 graded light levels, from 0.001 footlambert to 30,000 footlamberts. (The footlambert is a unit

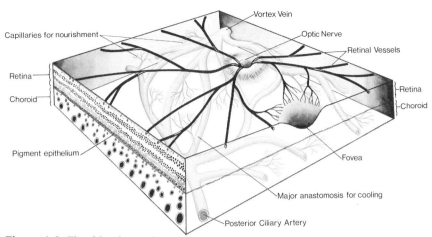

Figure 1-9. Fine blood-vessel system of the retina and the choroid. (Artist: Laurel Cook.)

of brightness equal to 10^{13} photons falling on an area of 1 cm² per second.) A comparison with the speeds of photographic film will provide a sense of just how extraordinary this range of sensitivity is. Most films range from ASA 50 (for bright light) to ASA 400 (for dim light). On the same scale the retina's sensitivity ranges from ASA 50 to ASA 5000.

Just as the retina is capable of great sensitivity, it is also capable of great discrimination. The human retina can perceive that two objects are two and not one when those two objects are separated by a space that subtends an angle of but five minutes of a degree. For example, at a distance of 20 feet (~6 m), the horizontal lines of a capital "E" need be separated from each other by only 1.8 mm in order to be perceived as distinct lines. A physical separation of objects of this magnitude would correspond to a separation of slightly greater than 0.001 mm (1.0 μm) on the retinal image. In contrast to this great ability to resolve detail is the 150°-wide field of view that the retina can record because of its hemispheric shape.

The retina continually records and erases its imagery, so that it is always ready for the next event. For example, an average reader can cover 250 words of this book in one minute. Since the foveal region of the retina can record an average of three words per glance, the average reader will make about 80 physiologic erasures per minute. Since storage time in the retina averages 0.1 second, a maximum of 600 physiologic erasures can, theoretically, be made every minute.

The retina is, however, capable of altering the length of its sampling time. With plenty of light available, the retina may take readings every 0.1 second. When the lighting is dim, the retina will integrate light from a scene for about 0.2 second. This effect will bring out fainter detail, but at the expense of perceiving less movement.

Photoreceptors. The receptor cells of the retina come in two varieties, and each has a different function. The *cones* record color vision, and are concentrated in the *macula,* the central 10° of the retina. Three types of cones with differing pigment compositions enable us to discern over 150 different colors and countless nuances of those colors. The central 2° of the macula is the *fovea* (Fig. 1-10), an area about 200 cones long by 200 cones wide and responsible for fine visual discrimination, such as reading fine print. Roughly 14% of the seven million cones are concentrated in the macula and fovea; the remainder are dispersed over the rest of the retina so that color can be appreciated over the entire visual field.[14]

The 123 million *rods* are the photoreceptors responsible for registering black, gray, and white impressions, and are also the sole means of sight in very dim light. Each rod contains 10 million molecules of a pigment known as *rhodopsin,* a complex molecule consisting of a vitamin A homologue and a protein. These molecules are stored on a stack of discs within the outer segment of the rod. Each day, the discs at the tip of the receptor are consumed by the pigment epithelium while new discs are added from below. It should be noted that cones also have stacks of photo pigment which are renewed daily. Light stimulates rhodopsin to undergo a series of chemical changes that ultimately result in triggering a nerve impulse to the brain. During a period when one's eyes are becoming accustomed to the dark, rhodopsin acts as a chemical amplifier, requiring about a half hour to become sensitive enough to sense just a few quanta of light. Substantial amplification must occur since the energy in one quantum of green light is about 4×10^{-12} ergs.

The rods and cones are linked into groups called *receptor fields.* The receptor fields of cones in the fovea are small and are organized so as to enhance the contrast of that part of the image that falls on them. Toward the periphery of the retina, the grouping into receptor fields becomes broader so that shapes can be recognized more easily in dim light.[15]

The rods and cones in the receptor fields convert the light energy that strikes them into chemoelectric impulses, the language of the nervous system. The impulses from the 130 million photoreceptors must be organized into meaningful patterns and condensed before they leave the retina through the one million optic-nerve fibers. The job of such condensation and grouping belongs to the cells that lie between the rods and cones, the *horizontal, bipolar,* and *amacrine cells.* The former two are nerve cells that serve the rods and cones; the latter is a modified nerve cell that possesses no long processes, as do other nerve cells. The nerve fibers serving these cells converge at the back of the eye to form the optic nerve (Fig. 1-11).

Blind Spot. There are no rods or cones where the nerve fibers converge and pass through the surface of the retina to form the optic nerve. This is the *blind spot,* and portions of the retinal image falling on

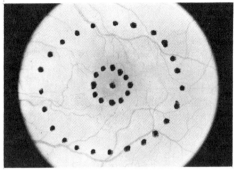

Figure 1-10. The area of the macula and fovea as seen with the ophthalmoscope. *Large circle:* macula outline. *Smaller circle:* fovea. *Central dot:* foveola.

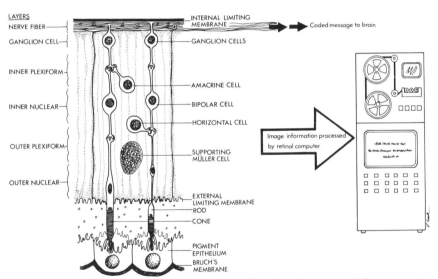

Figure 1-11. The retinal anatomy as seen under the microscope. The computer reminds us of all the information-processing done by the retina. (Artist: Laurel Cook.)

this area are not registered. We all have a blind spot, but it is generally not noticed unless it is mapped out by a physician in a visual-field examination. The blind spot is occasionally enlarged in hypertension, in advanced thyroid exopathalmos, or when pressure on the optic nerve from a brain tumor causes the optic nerve to swell and drape itself over the surrounding rods and cones.

Optic Nerve. The optic nerve functions as a telephone cable, bringing coded visual information to the brain. The optic nerve contains about a million nerve fibers, accompanying blood vessels and dividing septa, yet it measures only 1.5 mm in diameter. Its length in the orbit is 25 mm, with enough slack that it is never stretched during extreme eye rotation. It then runs 10 mm through the optic canal before it contacts the optic nerve from the other side in an area called the chiasm.

Pigment Epithelium. The *pigment epithelium* is the outermost layer of the retina and is adjoined by the choroid on the outside. Its cells contain pigment in order to absorb stray light, and they directly underlie the rods and the cones. They function to extract and deliver nutrients from the choroidal vascular network to the photoreceptors, and to collect and dispose of metabolic wastes from those same cells. Despite their close association and the great amount of activity that takes place between them, the photoreceptors and the pigment epithelium simply interdigitate in a mucopolysaccharide matrix. During life this connection is firm, but autopsy specimens show retinal separation from the pigment epithelium. There are only two limited areas of anatomic connection between them, the *ora serrata* and the *optic disc.*

The electron microscope reveals that the retina-pigment epithelium complex is very similar to the brain-choroid plexus epithelium complex. For example, both epithelia are joined by tight junctions that are effective barriers to the passage of ions between cells, and both epithelial surfaces face fenestrated choroid capillaries.

Blood Supply. Figure 1-9 presents a view of the arrangement of the large blood vessels within the retina, revealing the complicated interlacing net of capillaries that supply the retina. Although the vasculature in the retina is extensive, it cannot efficiently supply the retina's posterior layer, which contains the receptor cells, the rods, and the cones. These photosensitive elements are helped by the vessels of the choroid for their nutrition.

In a condition known as retinal detachment, a layer of fluid separates the retina from its underlying pigment epithelial layer. The area of separated retina functions very poorly until the retina is surgically reattached. Diabetic retinopathy results from another derangement of the retinal vasculature. It is discussed in Chapter 11.

Vitreous Humor

The *vitreous humor,* or vitreous, occupies four-fifths of the volume of the eyeball. It is not simply inert jelly, but has structure and a surrounding envelope (Figs. 1-12, 1-13).[16] Within the body of the vitreous, fine collagen fibers crisscross to form a scaffolding. The resulting matrix is filled with a viscous mucopolysaccharide, hyaluronic acid. The components of the vitreous are almost 99% water, and perfectly clear. Hyaluronic acid is a great shock absorber. If it is compressed slowly it rebounds

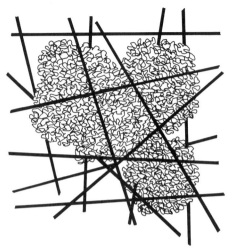

Figure 1-12. Microscopic anatomy of the vitreous showing spongy hyaluronic acid molecule between collagen fibers. (Courtesy of Dr. E.A. Balazs.)

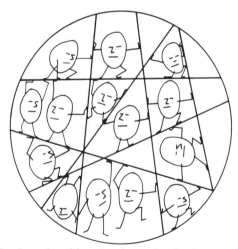

Figure 1-13. How hyaluronic acid molecules maintain the structural integrity of the vitreous. (Courtesy of Dr. E.A. Balazs.)

slowly, but when it is compressed rapidly, as when the eye is struck by a fast-moving squash ball, for example, the rebound is even faster than the compression.

The envelope surrounding the vitreous is primarily a condensate of the gel and is anchored to the more forward portion of the retina, the *ora serrata,* at the head of the optic nerve along the major retinal blood vessels, and in areas where retinal inflammation has occurred (Fig. 1-14). If the vitreous gel shrinks, the resulting tension on its anchors produces a tear in

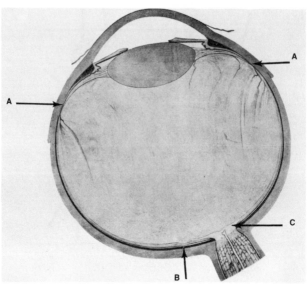

Figure 1-14. Normal attachment sites of the vitreous to the retina. **A** Ora serrata. **B** Macula. **C** Optic nerve.

the retina, which allows the adjacent vitreous to enter between the choroid and retina, producing retinal detachment.

With age, some of the collagen fibers of the vitreous often break away from the main superstructure. The free fibers may condense into balls or strands and float freely in watery pools that form in the vitreous. Patients with such changes often see floating specks or webs, which move as their eyes move and are mildly annoying but usually harmless, and which often disappear in time.

Sclera

The sclera (the "white" of the eye) is the eye's spherical, tough, outer layer, akin to tendon in structure. Continuous with the cornea, it is opaque, has a scanty superficial blood supply, and is very similar in microscopic structure to the cornea. The cornea is transparent and the sclera opaque because the collagen fibers making up the cornea are much finer and are arranged in a more orderly fashion than those of the sclera.

Conjunctiva

This clear membrane, with its almost invisible blood vessels, covers the sclera and also lines the inner surfaces of both upper and lower lids (Fig. 1-1). The role of the conjunctiva is to defend and repair the cornea in the event of scratches, wounds, or infections. The blood vessels of the conjunctiva dilate, leaking nutrients, antibodies, and leukocytes into the tears, which then wash over the avascular corneal surface. The conjunctiva also secretes mucus and oil, both of which help to keep the cornea moist and clean and to reduce friction when the lid blinks over the cornea.[17] The conjunctival mucus film over the ocular surface seems to catch microorganisms much as fly paper catches flies. This mucus net then condenses into a ball and is carried to the *nasal canthus* (inner corner of the eye) where it will dry out and roll onto the skin. Finally, the conjunctiva helps to resurface the cornea with epithelial cells should the entire corneal surface be scraped or burned.[18]

Orbit

The eyeball and its muscle and nerve attachments are packed in a fat-filled bony socket called the *orbit.* The orbital volume is about 30 cc, or that of a "shot" glass. The fat serves to provide almost frictionless movement of the eye. The paper-thin floor of the orbit, the *lamina papyracea,* is actually the roof of the maxillary sinus. Thus, in severe facial trauma, which often produces a gaping fracture of the orbital floor, the orbital fat or the inferior rectus muscle may fall into the crack, giving the eye a sunken appearance. Sometimes the inferior rectus may be caught in the fracture, restricting upward eye movement. Such a fracture is known as a "blowout fracture" of the orbit.

In surgical exploration of the orbit, the surgeon will bravely enter through the lateral wall. It is interesting to note that the distance from the anterior orbital rim to the middle cranial fossa, which holds the brain, is only 3 cm.

Lacrimal System

The lacrimal (tear) gland, nestled in the orbit just below the brow, and a tear drainage system constitute the lacrimal system. The drainage system consists of one small hole *(puncta)* in each lid that leads through a series of *lacrimal canaliculi* (small ducts) to the *lacrimal sac.* This sac, located near the inner corner of the eye, empties through the *nasolacrimal duct* into the *inferior meatus* of the nasal cavity, which drains into either the nares or the nasopharynx (Fig. 1-15). The tear gland produces about 0.2 ml of tears in a normal 24-hour day. After washing the cornea and conjunctiva, some of the tears evaporate, but most drain through the puncta down to the nose and into the throat.[17] In older people the delicate canaliculi and nasolacrimal ducts leading to the nose occasionally become plugged or kinked. Such patients complain of blurred vision and of constantly watering eyes. This annoying condition, although not serious, may be treated with local therapy for any condition that may be deforming the duct; more radical

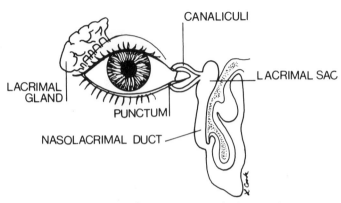

Figure 1-15. Lacrimal system anatomy. Tears drain out the upper and lower puncta via canaliculi and through the lacrimal sac to the back of the nose. (Artist: Laurel Cook.)

therapy may include mechanical dilation or surgical construction of a new artificial passageway. The latter operation creates a new channel from the corner of the eye to the nose.

Extraocular Muscles

The eyes can move in almost any direction at a variety of speeds through the coordinated effort of the six muscles attached to each eye. The muscles can also be thought of as stabilizing the eye in the orbit. Figure 1-16 depicts the placement of each of the *extraocular muscles* (EOM).

Since muscle actions actually change according to the position of the eye, the reader is referred to a neuroophthalmologic text for a more complete description of muscle action. Table 1-2 is, however, a helpful guide in becoming acquainted with the EOM.

Nerve and Brain Control. The *medical rectus, superior rectus, inferior rectus,* and *inferior oblique* muscles are commanded by the third cranial nerve. Damage to the brain stem, therefore, not only causes problems in some vital body function, but also may interfere with eye movement in certain directions.[19] Ultimately, the brain's frontal center and cerebellum are responsible for controlling eye movement.[20] In cerebellar disease, this control is sometimes deranged in such a way that the eyes will overshoot an object that they are turning to view. This condition is called *ocular dysmetria.*

Types of Eye Movement. Both eyes may move in opposite directions at the same time (e.g., both rotating toward the nose), as in *convergence* movement, or they may move in the same direction, as in comitant movement. There are two types of comitant movement, saccadic and

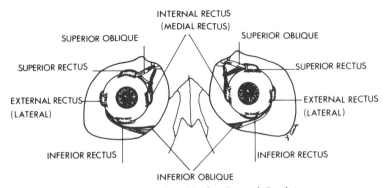

Figure 1-16. The extraocular muscles. (Artist: Laurel Cook.)

Table 1-2. Extrinsic Eye Muscles: Actions and Innervations

Muscle	Action	Cranial-Nerve Innervation
Superior rectus	Elevates the eye	III (Oculomotor)
Inferior rectus	Depresses eye	III (Oculomotor)
Medial rectus	Moves eye nasally (adduction)	III (Oculomotor)
Lateral rectus	Moves eye temporally (abduction)	VI (Abducens)
Superior oblique[a]	Moves eye down (abducts) to examiner	IV (Trochlear)
	Twists R eye clockwise	
	Twists L eye counterclockwise	
Inferior oblique	Moves eye up, twists eye outward	III (Oculomotor)

[a]Known as the "cheater muscle" because it moves the eye down and out during exams.

pursuit movements.[21,22] *Saccade* is an old French word meaning the flick of a sail. A saccadic movement is made when one catches a glimpse of a stranger out of the corner of the eye or when one looks for the source of a startling noise off to the side. These movements have a range of $1/4°$ to $90°$, and can be made in a fraction of a second with amazing accuracy. Such movements are used during reading. This system of movement is usually developed by three weeks of age. Pursuit movement is the type of smooth, controlled movement used to watch the continuous movement of a kite floating in the breeze. Under these circumstances, the eye and brain rapidly compute the speed of the kite, and continuously send the proper signals to the eye muscles to keep the kite focused on the fovea. In this system, the kite is always about ¹/₆ of a second ahead of the eye movement. If after a while, however, the kite were to sway back and forth in a regular fashion, the pursuit system could quickly learn to anticipate the next movement, and the small time lag might vanish. By age three months, infants have a working pursuit system.

Convergence movements, used to focus on a close object, are brought about by simultaneous activation of the medial recti muscles of both eyes. The convergence reflex works in conjunction with both the accommodation mechanism and pupillary constriction, and so, when the eyes converge a fixed number of degrees, the lens accommodates a corresponding fixed number of diopters and the pupil constricts a fixed number of millimeters. Each person is born with a unique set of accommodative-convergence-pupillary relationships, and the reflex remains constant throughout life until, with age, the lens begins to lose elasticity.

Eyelids

The eyelids are closed by an oval, three-part muscle *(orbicularis)* that primarily squeezes and twists the upper lid down while keeping the lower lid at a constant level. It is also noted that as either lid moves during the blink it twists nasally to improve tear flow. Acting in opposition to the orbicularis, the *levator* lifts the upper lid. (Orientals lack upper-lid folds because their levator muscles do not insert into the skin of the upper lids [Fig. 1-17]). We blink about four to six times a minute. When concentrating on a task, we may blink but once or twice a minute; when bored, 10 to 15 times a minute.

Drooping of the lid, *ptosis,* is often caused by a third cranial-nerve palsy. A turned-in lower lid *(entropion),* often seen in older people, allows the lashes to scratch the cornea. Conversely, a turned-out lid *(ectropion)* often causes disturbances in tear flow. Baggy lower lids occur often in older people and are due to orbital fat herniating through the orbital septum into the lower lid, a phenomenon called *blepharochalasis.* Xanthelasma is an elongated fatty yellow lesion that forms under the skin of the upper and lower lids. It is often hereditary, and roughly a third of the cases have a history of elevated serum lipids. The lesions are cosmetically ugly and simple to excise, but the patient should be warned that the lesions recur in about one-third of the cases and will have to be excised a second or even a third time.[23] In Bell's palsy, all muscles of an entire side of the face are paralyzed, and the eye on that side remains open because the orbicularis is unable to close it. Ironically, while the cornea dries, the absence of lid twist, a motion controlled by one of the subdivisions of the orbicularis, prevents tear pumping and tear drainage, and the lower eye

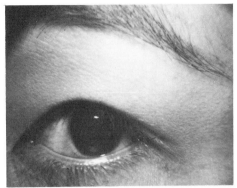

Figure 1-17. Mongolian lid. Note the absence of the usual upper-lid fold.

fills with tears. To prevent the cornea from drying out, the lid is usually taped or sewed shut until the paralysis disappears. Finally, upper eye lashes function as sunshades. One has only to see the long lashes of the giraffe, with its head high above the trees, to appreciate the role of the lashes as sunshades. The lower lashes may have been designed to wipe foreign bodies from the inner surface of the upper lid. Most children instinctively pull their upper lids down over the lower lashes in attempting to remove "something in their eye."

Eyebrows

Anatomically, the brow delineates the superior orbital rim. The brow seems to function primarily as a ledge that partially prevents forehead sweat from running into the eyes, and probably functions as a sunshade in keeping stray light from striking the cornea. For reasons poorly understood, brow and lash hair grow to a fixed length and usually stop. In the Trobriand and Marshall Bennet Islands, brows are chewed off as a sign of love, and Amazon maidens pluck out their brows to beautify themselves.[24] Interestingly, the outer third of the eyebrow often thins or disappears by itself in thyroid disease.

References

1. Vaughan HG, Schlimmel H: Feasibility of electrocortical visual prostheses. In: *Visual Prosthesis, The Interdisciplinary Dialogue.* Edited by RD Sterling, EA Bensig, SU Pollack, et al. New York, Academic Press, 1971, pp 65–79

2. Tolansky S: *Optical Illusions.* London, Pergamon, 1964, p 95

3. Hubel DH: The visual cortex of the brain. Sci Am 209:54, 1963

4. Valvro A: *Sight Restoration After Long-Term Blindness. The Problems and Behavior Patterns of Visual Rehabilitation.* New York, American Foundation for the Blind, 1971, pp 14–15

5. Goldman H: Studien veber den Alterskernstreifen der Linse. Arch Augenhelk 110:405, 1937

6. Alpern M: *Accommodation in the Eye,* Vol 3. Edited by H Dawson. New York, Academic Press, 1971, p 191

7. Fry EH, Hall-Parker JB: Eye hue and the oculocardiac reflex. Br J Ophthalmol 62:116, 1978

8. Wolff E: *The Anatomy of the Eye & Orbit.* New York, McGraw-Hill, 1951, p 70

9. Woodhouse JM, Campbell FW: The role of the pupil light reflex in aiding adaptation to the dark. Vision Res 15:649, 1975

10. Stark L: Stability, oscillations and noise in the human pupil servomechanism. Proc IRE 47:1925, 1959

11. Hess EH: Attitude and pupil size. Sci Am 212:46, 1965

12. Fisher RF: The force of contraction of the human ciliary muscle during accommodation. J Physiol 270:51, 1977

13. Hayreh SS: Choroidal circulation in health and in acute vascular occlusion. In: *Vision and Circulation.* Edited by JS Cant. St. Louis, Mosby, 1976, pp 157–170

14. Gregory RL: *Eye and Brain.* New York, McGraw-Hill, 1966, pp 34–116

15. Glezer VD: The receptive fields of the retina. Vision Res 5:497, 1961

16. Balazs EA: Molecular morphology of the vitreous body. In: *The Structure of the Eye.* Edited by GK Smelser. New York, Academic Press, 1961, p 293

17. Holly FJ, Lemp MA: The precorneal tear film and dry eye syndromes. Int Ophthalmol Clin 13:108, 1973

18. Friedenwald JS: Growth pressure and metaplasia of conjunctival and corneal epithelium. Documenta Ophthalmol 184:5, 1951

19. Wolff E: *The Anatomy of the Eye and Orbit.* New York, McGraw-Hill, 1951, pp 201–222

20. Bach-y-Rita, Collins CC: *The Control of Eye Movements.* New York, Academic Press, 1971, pp 429, 447

21. Robinson D: The mechanics of human saccadic eye movement. J Physiol 174:245, 1964

22. Miller D: Saccadic and pursuit systems: a review. J Pediatr Ophthalmol 5:39, 1968

23. Mendelson BC, Masson JK: Xanthelasma: followup on results after surgical excision. Plast Reconstr Surg 58:535, 1976

24. Mann I: *Culture, Race, Climate and Eye Disease.* Springfield, Ill, Thomas, 1961, pp 47–61

Chapter 2

Testing

When we look at the eyes, we as human beings instinctively look for meaning, not anatomic detail. Eyes portray happiness, anger, suspicion, surprise, and grief. Yet the observant physicians must erase their instinctive recognition of the eye as an emotional transmitter and look at the eyes and lids in an unemotional and analytical manner.

The use of a mnemonic device, i.e., the word PUPIL, will help one develop a systematic approach to examination and illustrate the self-revealing nature of many eye problems. Thus, in examining the ophthalmologic patient, the physician might proceed from P through L of the system as follows:

P—Position of eyes (Are they bulging, sunken, cross-eyed, wall-eyed?)
U—Upper and lower lids
P—Pupils (What are their sizes, shapes, and reactions to light, black, and gray?)
I—Inflammation (Is there redness of conjunctiva? What is the distribution of redness?)
L—Luster (Is the cornea shiny? Is your flashlight's reflection round and smooth, or irregular? Is the cornea clear or gray?)

Figures 2-1 through 2-8 are photos of some common eye abnormalities. As an exercise, the student may wish to study each case by using this mnemonic device, to observe for himself how straightforward the diagnosis can be.

Symptoms

Consider how many questions a wise internist must ask of a patient before he might even suspect that the patient's problem is a diseased liver or

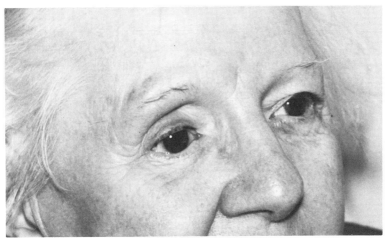

Figure 2-1. Right-eye ocular prosthesis (note deep lid fold); the patient complained of burning eyes. (Courtesy of Raymond Jahrling.)

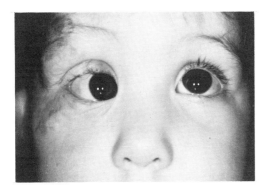

Figure 2-2. Right esotropia (note light reflection near limbus). The patient's mother reported double vision and an abnormal appearance of the lid.

pancreas. This need not be the case in ophthalmologic practice. These patients usually are able to tell you at once that their eyes hurt or that they cannot see. Once you are given the lead, your job is to decide which part of the eye is abnormal.

If the chief complaint is eye pain, for instance, you must know that pain can originate from the following structures:

1. Conjunctiva

2. Cornea

3. Iris and ciliary body

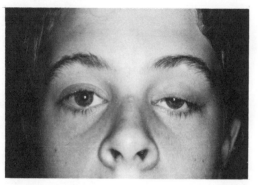

Figure 2-3. Right ptosis of the lid. The patient complained of a drooping lid. (Courtesy of Dr. Arthur S. Grove.)

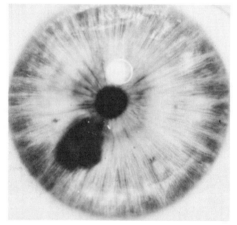

Figure 2-4. Iris nevus. The patient had reported for a routine eye examination.

4. Orbital structures (optic nerves)

5. Paranasal sinuses

Thus, your testing would revolve around analyzing these parts. If the eye pain is associated with increased light sensitivity, you must know that only the following structures can be diseased:

1. Cornea

2. Iris and ciliary body

3. Optic nerve

If the eye is tender when gently pressed through the upper lid, you might reduce the possibilities to diseases of the optic nerve and the iris and

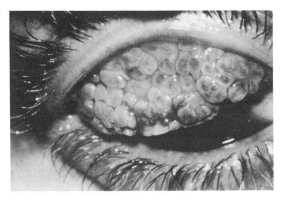

Figure 2-5. Vernal conjunctivitis (follicles on everted lid surface). The patient complained of eye irritation. (Courtesy of American Academy of Ophthalmology.)

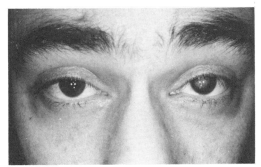

Figure 2-6. Mature cataract (left eye). The patient complained of poor vision.

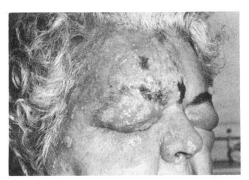

Figure 2-7. Herpes zoster dermatitis on the left eye. The patient complained of eye irritation and light sensitivity. (Courtesy of Dr. Kenneth Arndt.)

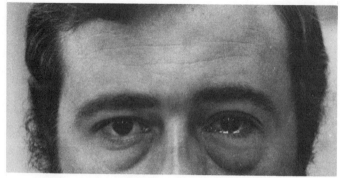

Figure 2-8. Cystic swelling of the left lid (allergy). The patient complained of swelling and itchiness of both lids.

ciliary body. If the pain is more severe when the eyes move, you might conclude that optic-nerve inflammation is present.

Aside from pain, the other major eye complaint is poor vision. You must first decide if this is due to organic disease or to refractive error (myopia, astigmatism, hyperopia, presbyopia). Most organic diseases have a relatively acute onset, i.e., days to months, whereas refractive errors are usually present for years. Use of the pinhole in testing visual acuity—discussed in the next section—is a quick way to differentiate refractive errors from organic eye disease.

Once refractive error is ruled out, the cause of loss of vision can be narrowed to trouble in one of the following structures:

1. Cornea

2. Lens

3. Iris and ciliary body

4. Vitreous

5. Retina

6. Optic nerve

7. Brain

Except for the brain, all of these structures can be seen and inspected with some form of examining equipment. An exception would be a transitory embolus, which interferes with retinal circulation for 15 to 30 minutes and then disappears with no trace, or with a trace in the form of a cholesterol plaque stuck in one of the small capillary channels.

History

Past Illness or Surgery

Diabetes, hypertension, rheumatoid arthritis, neurologic disease, and brain tumors all affect vision. The physician must therefore determine whether the patient has ever had any of these systemic conditions. He must also ask specifically whether the patient has had any eye operation or severe injury.

Allergies

Since you may be putting certain drops in the eye, or prescribing certain medications, it is very important that you ask if the patient is allergic to any medications.

Use of Medications

Is the patient taking any systemic medications or eyedrops now? For example, you should know that

1. Chloroquine can cause blurring of vision due to retinal pathology

2. Ethambutol can cause inflammation of the optic nerve

3. Chloromycetin® can cause optic neuritis from prolonged therapy

4. Corticosteroids can produce cataracts and glaucoma

5. Phenothiazine tranquilizers can cause pigmentary retinopathy.[1]

Family History

Because the possibility of hereditary disease must be considered, the patient should be questioned about blindness or any eye surgery in other family members. Specifically, the physician should know of any hereditary predispositions to glaucoma, cataracts, macular degeneration, or crossed eyes.

Testing Vision

Distance Vision

Not too long ago, the scrub nurse in our operating room was preparing the instrument table for an operation. One of the very fine sutures, with the needle attached, fell onto the black-and-white checkered floor by accident. As I walked into the room, she was on her hands and knees looking for the suture and needle. How futile, I thought, to look for something so fine on such a confusing background. All at once she stopped, reached down, and came up grinning with the suture. "What amazing eyesight!" I exclaimed. Not long after this episode, she came into the eye clinic for a routine checkup. When we flashed the Snellen chart on the wall, she could read no better than 20/100. She was nearsighted, and only after getting the proper glasses could she see 20/20. Yet, under my very eyes, this nurse had performed a visual miracle in the operating room. What then is good vision?

The nurse, a myope, would not be considered to have good vision. By definition, good vision is distance vision measured on a test chart 20 feet from the patient. When we record a patient's vision, we are actually comparing it with a man from Utrecht, Holland, back in 1864. At that time, Professor Herman Snellen, later to be Chief of Ophthalmology at Utrecht, was preoccupied with the task of quantifying visual acuity. His assistant was a man who seemed to see better than anyone else at the hospital. When Professor Snellen designed his charts of variously sized letters, he always compared the patient's visual performance at 20 feet with that of his assistant. Thus, if a patient read a line designated 20/40, it meant that the patient saw at 20 feet what Professor Snellen's assistant saw at 40 feet. Vision of 20/200, of course, meant that the patient saw 20 feet away what the assistant could read at 200 feet (Fig. 2-9).[2]

Upon closer analysis, the Snellen system, which is empirical, closely agrees with predictable optic principles. Professor Snellen's assistant could really identify the key parts of any letter if the retinal image of the key parts were separated by the width of a retinal cone (1 micron), or one minute of arc. Thus, at a testing distance of 10 meters (33 feet), the bars of the "E" would have to be spaced 3 mm apart, at 6 meters (20 feet) they would be spaced at 1.8 mm, and at 60 meters (200 feet) they would be spread by 18 mm. Occasionally, the patient cannot see even the largest letter on the chart (usually the 20/200 letter). Customarily, the examiner will hold up 2 or 3 fingers from across the room and slowly walk to the patient until the patient can identify the number of fingers held up. Thus visual acuity might be recorded as CF (counting fingers) at 4 feet or CF at 6 inches in more severe cases. If vision is so impaired that the number of fingers of the examiner is not identifiable, then the patient is asked if he or she can see the hand of the examiner move. Such vision is recorded as HM (hand movement) vision. If such movement cannot be discerned, the patient is asked whether a flashlight is held above or below the patient's eye, and the direction of the light is registered. If this can be done, the patient is said to have accurate light projection. If the patient cannot discern the direction of the light, but *can* perceive the light, he or she is said to have light perception (LP).

To sum up, the Snellen chart is used to test visual acuity of from

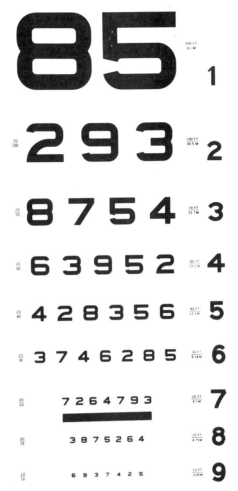

Figure 2-9. The Snellen chart.

20/20 to 20/200 or 20/400 (depending on the chart used), then CF (distance of identification), HM, accurate light projection, LP (light perception), and, finally, NIL (no vision).

In a routine eye exam, be sure to record the patient's visual acuity for legal purposes, as well as for establishing a baseline before performing other tests.

Always record the visual acuity with the patient's glasses on. Remember, organic trouble or refractive error can diminish visual acuity. If visual acuity is recorded with glasses on, and vision is diminished, either the glasses are no longer adequate or an organic disease is present. If the glasses are new, the problem is probably organic. What if the glasses are old, or the patient has lost his glasses? Is there a way to rule out refractive problems? *The pinhole test!* Hold up a piece of cardboard with a pinhole in the center, or purchase a professional, black plastic pinhole occluder. Whichever you use, if the patient's vision improves significantly with the pinhole, the problem is most likely refractive. Certainly a lens, retinal, or optic-nerve problem would not abate significantly with a simple pinhole.

The Snellen chart itself comes in two basic forms. The inexpensive cardboard form is placed 20 feet from the patient and is illuminated by a 100-watt bulb directed toward the chart. The second type, a projector with a Snellen chart slide, is presented in a darkened room. The projector automatically gives a calibrated illumination and has the capacity to isolate single letters or lines.

Near Vision

Near vision becomes a problem in people over 45 years of age when accommodative power has waned, and it becomes difficult to see newsprint held 33 cm (or 13 inches) from the eyes. This task requires about 3 D of accommodation (100 ÷ 33 cm = 3 D) and, unfortunately, the 15 D of accommodation given to us at birth has shrunken to less than 3 D by the time we reach age 45.

To measure near visual acuity, Dr. Edward Jaeger, a Viennese ophthalmologist, developed a near reading chart composed of variously sized letters using ordinary printer's type.[3] This chart helps to determine one's visual threshold for a near task and then helps to document the degree of improvement after the proper reading glasses have been prescribed. Since Professor Jaeger's chart was first developed, different notations for the variously sized print on the near-reading chart have been proposed. Table 2-1 shows the different notations for letters of the

Table 2-1. Jaeger Notations for Near-Vision Testing with Snellen Equivalents

Jaeger	*20/20 System*	*14-Inch System*
J1	20/20	14/14
J3	20/30	14/21
J5	20/40	14/28
J6	20/50	14/35
J7	20/60	14/42
J9	20/85	14/64
J11	20/120	14/79
J12	20/130	14/89

same size. On the left is the "J," or Jaeger, notation. In the center column, the equally sized letters have been mathematically converted into the conventional Snellen 20/20 system, which really uses the minimum angle appreciated between identifiable parts of a letter. On the right is a modified Snellen system based on a distance of 14 inches. *Remember, use a good reading light when testing near vision.*

Visual Field

The Snellen chart measures *foveal vision,* which encompasses the central 2° of our visual world, but what about the rest of the field of view, which amounts to about 150°? Certain authorities refer to all vision outside the central few degrees as *side,* or *peripheral, vision,* or as the patient's visual field.

A portion of the visual field can be missing if a portion of the retina is diseased, as occurs in a partially detached retina (Fig. 2-10). A field defect can also occur if some of the fibers of the optic nerve have been destroyed, as in glaucoma (Fig. 2-11), or if some of the visual fibers passing through the brain are pinched, and sometimes permanently destroyed, by a tumor of the pituitary gland. Figure 2-12 shows a characteristic bitemporal temporal-field defect caused by tumor compression of the decussating fibers in the optic chiasm. As a matter of fact, there is a popular medical interpretation of David's biblical victory over the Philistine giant, Goliath. The theory holds that Goliath was a giant because of an abnormal production of growth hormone, secreted by the wild cells of a pituitary gland tumor. The tumor had pressed on the visual fibers of the optic chiasm, destroying those representing Goliath's side vision. David sensed that the giant had a blind side, and so was able to approach from that side, getting close enough to deliver the fatal blow with his sling.

During the end of the nineteenth century, Dr. Bjerrum, Professor of Ophthalmology at Copenhagen, discovered that he could plot an accurate visual field on a large black cloth stretched over a pair of large doors in his office.[4] During the test a weak light illuminated the cloth, and the patient was asked to concentrate on a small button sewn on the center. Since one eye can often compensate for a blind area in the other eye, one eye was always covered while the field of the second eye was plotted. Once assured that the patient's eye was fixed on the screen's center, Dr. Bjerrum brought in a small white target from the side and asked the patient to report when it became visible. If a blind area were picked up, its limits were plotted by moving the target away from the blind area until the patient noted its presence.

The amount of time needed for this test varies from 3 to 30 minutes, depending on the examiner's expertise and on the patient's ability to concentrate. Since the exam can be time-consuming, it has been recommended for use only in the following situations:

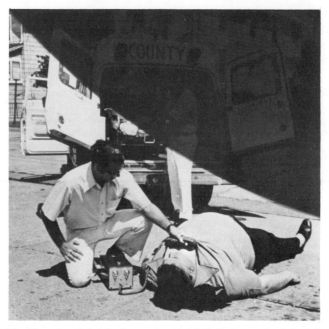

Figure 2-10. The visual field of a patient with inferior retinal detachment. The location of the field defect is the inverse of the location of the disease. (Courtesy of *Medical Data and Electronics*, Pittsburgh: Cover, Sept–Oct 1974.)

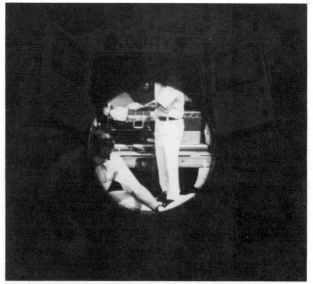

Figure 2-11. The visual field of one eye of a patient with advanced glaucoma. (Courtesy of *Medical Data and Electronics*, Pittsburgh.)

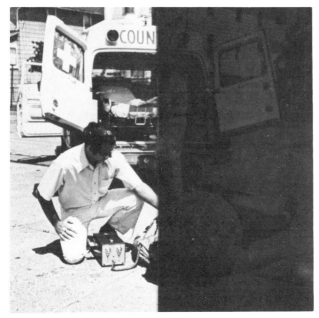

Figure 2-12. The visual field of one eye of a patient with a pituitary tumor (temporal hemianopia). (Courtesy of *Medical Data and Electronics,* Pittsburgh.)

1. When central vision is not correctable to 20/20 and a thorough eye examination reveals no obvious reason for the lowered vision

2. When the patient has known or suspected brain disease

3. When the patient has unexplained headaches

4. In the presence of a hemiparesis

5. In the presence of a swollen optic nerve (papilledema) as determined by ophthalmoscopic examination

6. When the patient has endocrine disturbances

7. When the patient has glaucoma

8. When the patient has difficulty seeing and avoiding obstacles in his path.

Central Visual-Field Examinations (Tangent-Screen Examination). As seen in Figure 2-13, the typical test uses a black felt screen illuminated by a weak bulb (7–10 W). The patient is seated 1 m from the screen, which allows the physician to plot the central 30°. A perimeter is used to plot the additional 120°. With one eye covered and prescribed distance-spectacles on the eyes, a large (try 9 mm) white test object at the end of a wand is

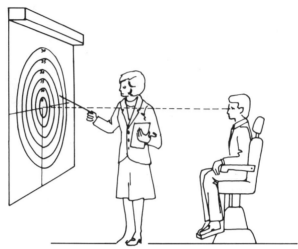

Figure 2-13. Examination of the central field with a Bjerrum (Tangent) Screen. (Artists: David Lobel and Laurel Cook.)

moved toward the center of the screen; if the patient performs well with this, the test is done with a 3 mm white test object. The patient is told to look at the central fixation target and to say "yes" when he sees a white spot coming in from the side. Seeing the wand, but not the white spot, does *not* call for an affirmative answer. The blind spot is usually mapped out at the beginning of the test by using a felt marking pencil or a set of black pins.

Sometimes tangent-screen results do not agree with a patient's everyday performances. We recently examined a patient whose test results showed that she had tunnel vision, i.e., she reported seeing only the central 5° of the screen. If these test results were accurate, this patient should have displayed severe problems with object avoidance, but when the lights were lowered and she was asked to navigate from one side of the room to the other, she deftly avoided all chairs and other obstacles in her path. In her case, therefore, the tangent-screen test results were inaccurate, and her condition probably represented a case of hysterical blindness.

Perimetry. Figure 2-14 displays a patient being tested in a perimeter. Such a device primarily measures the extent of the visual field in all meridians. Although it can plot the blind spot and blind areas within the central 30°, it does not provide the same magnified detail of these areas as the tangent-screen test.

Color Vision

Color blindness, or Daltonism, was named after John Dalton, the man who formulated the first practical atomic theory.[5] When we say that John

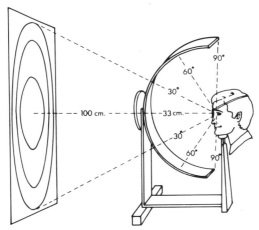

Figure 2-14. An illustration of the arc perimeter and the projection of the central 30° of the visual field chart. (Artists: David Lobel and Laurel Cook.)

Dalton was color blind, we do not mean that Dalton's visual world was made up of only blacks and whites and grays. We mean, rather, that he might wear a green vest instead of a red vest with his olive trousers. Most people who are color blind simply cannot distinguish between certain hues that are relatively close to each other in the visual spectrum. For example, a person with normal color vision can appreciate the difference between about 150 different pure colors, but a person with red-green confusion—the most common form of anomalous color vision—may see all the subtle differences in the blue end of the spectrum while differentiating very few colors in the red end, confusing greens, yellows, and reds. By utilizing various brightnesses and colors, it is possible to choose at least nine different colors that even the "color deficient" person will not confuse. It is likely that this principle was adopted to code medical gas cylinders, after a tragedy in which a color-deficient anesthetist gave carbon dioxide gas (from a green cylinder) instead of oxygen to a patient under anesthesia.

Interestingly, color blindness occurs much less often in certain peoples. Eskimos have a 0.8% incidence and Navajo's a 1.1% incidence, while white North Americans have an 8.4% incidence.[6] This phenomenon may be related to the process of natural selection and the survival value inherent in the ability to discriminate reds from greens, particularly dark reds from dark greens. Blood stains on the leaves of the forest floor, for instance, are the major means of stalking wounded prey. Oddly enough, the mammals that primitive man stalked (aside from the primates) do not have color vision.

Color blindness is also primarily a disease of men. Very few women have this problem. Females escape because they possess two X-chromosomes, which carry the genes for color vision, and only one of these chromosomes need be normal for normal color vision. Since the male has only one X-chromosome, a defect in it must produce whichever type of color vision it carries. The defect ultimately seems to reside in the cones of the retina. There are three different types of cones, each sensitive to almost all wavelengths of light, but one that is primarily sensitive to red, one to green, and one to blue. Therefore, a subtle deficiency in the red cone will lead to mild problems in any discrimination involving red. A more major deficiency in the red cone will lead to major mistakes in discriminating yellow-green from orange.

The various color tests try to determine (1) which cone type is deficient and (2) what degree of deficiency is present.

Protanopia and *protanomalous* refer to severe and mild red-cone problems, respectively. These patients confuse reds and greens.

Deuteranopia and *deuteranomalous* refer to severe and mild green-cone problems. These patients have another type of red-green confusion.

Tritanopia and *tritanomalous* refer to severe and mild blue-cone problems. This last type is very rare. These patients have trouble with blues and yellows.

The most commonly used color tests are the Ishihara Color Plates, the American Optical H-R-R Plates, and the Tokyo Medical College Plates. All are pictures consisting of letters or figures formed by small dots against a background of variously colored dots. The colors of the figures and background are designed to fall within the color confusion zones of people with color deficiencies.

Unfortunately, the color test plates are not sensitive enough to pick up a second type of color deficiency, *acquired color deficiency,* which is much rarer than the inherited type.[7] This second type is caused by disease of the retina or optic nerve. In general, diseases affecting the ganglion-cell layer of the retina and the fibers of the optic nerve, such as optic neuritis and tobacco- or alcohol-induced damage to the optic nerve, induce a red-green deficiency.

Such conditions as diabetic retinopathy, or toxicity from drugs like chloroquine and the phenothiazines, interfere with retinal function and usually produce a blue-yellow discrimination problem. There are practical problems in these situations, as indicated by the case of a patient with diabetic retinopathy who lost his ability to check his daily urine specimen for sugar by using a color-sensitive paper (Clinitest®).[8] In some patients overdosed with digitalis, everything appears yellow. One possible explanation might be that the metabolism of the blue cone is poisoned. Absence of a blue influence makes yellow stronger and the world takes on a yellow tinge.

To diagnose the acquired type of color deficiency, one must use a sophisticated test, such as the *D-5 test,* in which the subject must arrange 15 color discs from blue to red in proper spectral order. A similar test consisting of 100 colored discs would provide more precise testing.

From a practical point of view, a color-defective person should avoid a number of careers that demand good color discrimination, including navigation, traffic control, electrical work, and police work.[8]

Other Examination Techniques

Stereopsis

Because the interpupillary distance in adult humans averages 65 mm, the two eyes receive somewhat different views of the same object. In a process known as stereopsis, the brain takes the slightly different images from each eye and creates a three dimensional impression, giving a visual richness to the objects surrounding us. If the external muscles of both eyes are not working together perfectly, stereopsis cannot be achieved.

The simplest way to measure stereopsis, and thus the patient's degree of binocular function, is to place a pencil in each hand of the patient, and ask him to extend both hands forward and then to move the pencils toward each other until the tips touch (Fig. 2-15). It is impossible to get to touch both tips unless both eyes are open and working together.

How important is stereopsis in everyday life? One-eyed people certainly learn to make accurate depth judgments. A young patient of ours lost the sight of his right eye from a tree-branch laceration. Four months later he proved that he had regained a sense of depth, leading his Little League baseball team in hitting. There probably are, however, situations (albeit rare) in which shadows, or clues of movement, are not available to help him decide how far away an object is. Scientifically, stereoscopic acuity is described as the minimal detectible distance that one target can be appreciated to be in front of the second. One can also evaluate stereopsis by measuring the angles of rotation as the eyes move from a near object to a far object. The normal threshold of stereopsis in such cases is an angle of 10 to 40 minutes of arc.

Direct Ophthalmoscopy

Not too long ago a scientist from a flashbulb manufacturing company came to us with a problem. The company had designed a flashbulb which fitted directly into a small flat camera. Unfortunately, the subjects in all close-up pictures had red pupils (known as red eye in the camera industry). Optically speaking, this occurs when the axis of the light source and the viewing system of the camera are very close. The redness in the pupil actually is a somewhat unfocused image of the blood vessels in the choroid. In essence the flashbulb and flat camera combined to closely approximate the optics of the most important diagnostic instrument in eye work, the ophthalmoscope.

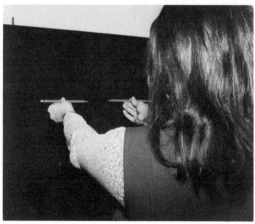

Figure 2-15. Testing for stereopsis using the pencil-tip-touch method.

The ophthalmoscope was discovered in 1851 by a 29-year-old physiologist named Helmholtz.[9] Four years previously, a well-known Viennese physiologist by the name of Ernst Brucke had reported noticing the red light in the pupil of a young man standing in the auditorium of the university when the direction of the chandelier light that reflected from the student's eye coincided with his own visual axis. Helmholtz explained his discovery in a letter to his father:

I had to explain to my students that the theory of emission of reflected light from the eye was discovered by Brucke. He was a hair's breath from the invention of the ophthalmoscope. He failed to ask himself what optical image was formed by the rays reflected from the luminous eye. . . .

To obtain an optical image of the retina, he had only to devise an instrument in which his eye could be placed in line with rays of light entering and leaving the observed eye.[10]

Helmholtz's invention became popular immediately. By 1855, pigmented retinopathy and detached retina, as well as the destruction of the optic nerve by glaucoma, had been seen and described. Thus an entire spectrum of blinding diseases could be understood and investigations of their causation and treatment could begin.

Figure 2-16 shows the way in which an ophthalmoscope works. It has its own light source, a viewing system, and a wheel of lenses that corrects the combined refractive errors of the examiner and patient. An understanding of this design principle allowed the camera manufacturer to solve his problem by elevating the flash cube just a few inches above the lens, thus moving it away from the optical axis of the lens.

In using the ophthalmoscope, a system of observation should be adopted. First turn the lens wheel to a +12.00. Hold the instrument about 10 cm from the eye. You are now focused on the cornea and lens.

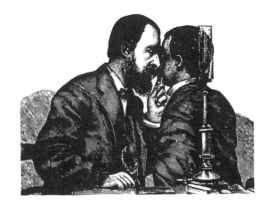

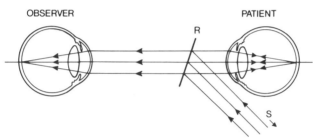

Figure 2-16. Direct ophthalmoscopy. *Top:* positioning patient. *Bottom:* optics.

Opacities of the cornea or lens will look black against an orange background.

Next, move closer to the patient's eye, keeping your eye at the viewing aperture and your index finger on the lens wheel. Get the optic disc in focus. Notice its color, margins (sharp or blurry), and the blood vessels coming from the disc, and finally ask the patient to look at your light. Now the macula is directed at you, and the glistening central dot is the fovea.

Pupil Dilation

The question often arises as to when to enlarge the pupil with drops prior to an ophthalmoscopic examination. Rather than listing the indications, it may be simpler to describe the contraindications:

1. Since most dilating drops blur the vision to some degree, do not dilate if the patient plans to drive himself home after the examination. Arrange a visit when a friend or family member will be able to drive the patient home.

2. If the patient has had a cataract extraction combined with an intraocular lens implantation, pupil dilation may dislocate the new lens. (See Chapter 8 for a discussion of this topic.)

3. If the patient has a neurologic problem, obtain the neurologist's permission before dilating the pupil. In certain cases of head trauma, the neurologist will want to follow pupil size for 24 to 48 hours, and dilation drops will interfere with this test.

4. If the anterior chamber looks shallow, or if there is a history of glaucoma in the family, try to see the optic nerve without pupil dilation. If this proves impossible, use a fast-acting mydriatic like 0.5% tropicamide (Mydriacyl®) or an easily reversed mydriatic like 10% phenylephrine.

Mydriatic drops have been known to precipitate an attack of angle-closure glaucoma, but how great is the risk in administering mydriatic eyedrops? Glaucoma affects about 2% of people over 40 years of age; of these about 5% have the angle-closure type of glaucoma. Angle-closure glaucoma is rare in people under 40 and reaches a peak incidence in people around 70 years old. Moreover, precipitation of angle-closure by mydriasis will occur in about 50% of those patients predisposed to the disease. Thus angle-closure glaucoma from pupil dilation should occur in less than one patient in a thousand over 40 years of age.

Indirect Ophthalmoscopy

The indirect ophthalmoscope allows the examiner to see more of the retina at one glance than does the direct ophthalmoscope. Because of its construction, this instrument accommodates a larger and brighter light source, which often allows the examiner to penetrate moderate cataracts in order to see retinal detail. Usually, however, the pupil must be dilated to use this device.

The indirect ophthalmoscope was invented by Dr. C. G. T. Reuter only one year after Helmholtz's invention of the direct scope.[10] The true usefulness of the device was not fully exploited, however, until 1947, when Dr. Charles Schepens of Boston modified it so that a stereoscopic view of the retina could be obtained at a comfortable viewing distance and so that the outer periphery of the retina could be visualized.[11] This was important because retinal tears that produce retinal detachments are usually located in the retinal periphery. Figure 2-17 shows the head-mounted scope of Dr. Schepens.

The indirect ophthalmoscope demands a great deal of practice before it can be used. The practice is well worth the time, because the skill afforded by such practice allows you to see the 3-dimensional elevation of the optic nerve in papilledema, shows the depths of the optic nerve in advanced glaucoma, gives a better perspective in a disseminated condition such as diabetic retinopathy, and is mandatory for evaluating a detached retina and for diagnosing a choroidal melanoma.

The indirect scope is used with three different lenses. The 14-D lens

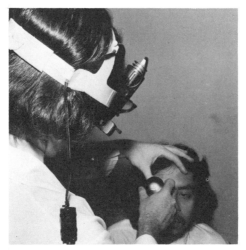

Figure 2-17. Head-mounted indirect ophthalmoscope.

gives a 4× magnification and a smaller field of view; the 30-D lens, a 2× magnification and the largest field; and the 20-D lens is a compromise between the other two. The *fundus* (or retinal) camera can be thought of simplistically as an enclosed indirect ophthalmoscope with a camera back.

Slit-Lamp Examination

The crystal on a watch appears relatively clear, and yet a penlight directed obliquely at the edge of the crystal brings out scratches and smears not easily seen in normal lighting. Similarly, the cornea, anterior chamber, lens, vitreous, and retina are clear tissues. They are not, however, perfectly transparent. In fact, such tissues backscatter 10% to 25% of the light that strikes them. Allivor Gullstrand of Stockholm, who won the Nobel prize in 1911 for his studies on the optics of the eye, realized that a very special system was needed to see structural detail in these so-called transparent tissues. Despite Gullstrand's use of a newly developed high-intensity light bulb, his new lamp still yielded poor resolution of ocular detail. To intensify the light further, he introduced a system of lenses that focused a fine slit of light sharply onto the cornea from an oblique direction. Gullstrand then added a modified microscope through which the illuminated structures could be seen. Finally, chin and forehead rests were added to stabilize the patient (Fig. 2-18).

The slit lamp is the backbone of the ophthalmologic examination. Like most sensitive instruments, it takes years of practice to become expert in its use. The slit lamp is used to evaluate corneal disease, characteristics of tears, types of cataracts, the postoperative course of many eye operations, inflammation of anterior chamber, and subtle

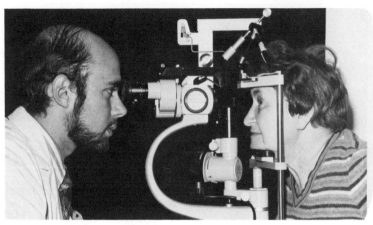

Figure 2-18. Slit-lamp examination.

conjunctival abnormalities. In conjunction with the applanation tonometer, it is used to record intraocular pressure; and in conjunction with various auxiliary lenses, it is used to evaluate the angle, the vitreous, the retina, and the optic nerve.

Tonometry

Since most patients with glaucoma are unaware that the pressure in the eye is abnormally elevated, some way had to be found to measure intraocular pressure. The device currently used to measure intraocular pressure is the indentation tonometer. Recently, a retired engineer asked to see the device after it had been applied to his eyes. His comment was, "We used to use the same thing to measure the sponginess of rubber. The softer the rubber, the deeper the indentation of the device, and the higher the reading on the scale." According to the same principle, Hjalmar August Schiotz developed a clinical indentation tonometer in 1905.[12] Because the tonometer must be placed on the cornea, a very sensitive tissue, accurate indentation tonometry is impossible without good corneal anesthesia. Thus, the tonometer could not have become a reality before 1884, when cocaine drops were introduced into ophthalmology.

Since 1905 a number of sophisticated and more accurate tonometers have been developed (Fig. 2-19), but for reasons of economy and simplicity, the Schiotz tonometer is the most widely used.

The procedures for Schiotz tonometry will not be described here. The procedures, although conceptually simple, should be learned under supervision (Fig. 2-20).

The contraindications for performing tonometry are corneal or conjunctival infection, corneal injury, or marked corneal distortion, i.e., conical or badly scarred corneas prevent accurate readings. For a more

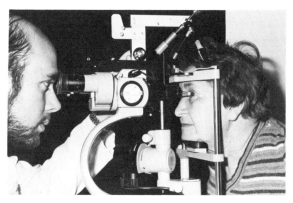

Figure 2-19. Applanation tonometer used with a slit lamp.

accurate measure of intraocular pressure, the ophthalmologist often uses the applanation tonometer (Fig. 2-20). Attached to the slit lamp and under microscopic control, this device records the pressure of the eye as the cornea is flattened in a very precise manner.

Exophthalmometry

As a gas station attendant fills the gasoline tank, the floating indicator is pushed up and this movement is registered on the gas gauge. In a similar manner, a tumor within the bony orbit pushes the eye out. Thus, by measuring the eye's protrusion, one can measure the tumor's growth. Since most orbital growths and tumors involve only one eye, measurement of the protrusion (or *proptosis*) of one eye, as compared to the normal eye, is known as *relative exophthalmometry.* Looking at the head in profile, the physician takes a measure (in millimeters) between the lateral rim of the orbit and the tip or apex of the cornea. The simplest way of making such a measurement is to hold a ruler along the side of the head and try to line up the edge of the lateral orbit and the cornea. A more precise device was designed in 1905 by Hertel, which still remains the most popular method of exophthalmometry.[13] The device is applied to the front of the face, like a pair of spectacles, and adjusted to the width of the head in order to tightly engage each orbital rim. Two mirrors with rulers angled at 45° are attached to each side of the exophthalmometer so that the examiner sees the eyes in profile, even though he or she is facing the patient. Measurement consists of lining up the corneal apex with the ruler.

In the case of a patient with a glioma of the right optic nerve, the reading might be:

O.D. 24 mm at 102 mm
O.S. 17 mm

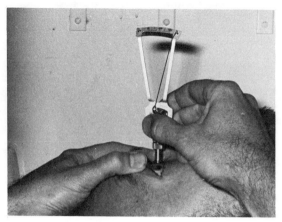

Figure 2-20. Indentation (Schiotz) tonometer poised over the patient's eye.

This means that the right corneal apex is 24 mm in front of the right orbital rim, the left corneal apex is 17 mm in front of the left orbital rim, and the exophthalmometer was set at a width of 102 mm. Thus, for consistency, all further measurements of this patient should be made at the same width.

The normal range of readings lie between 18 mm–24 mm, and a difference of 2 mm or more between both eyes is considered abnormal. In the case of Graves disease, one or both eyes may protrude beyond 24 mm.[14]

Gonioscopy

A goniometer is used by the scientist to measure angles; *gonioscopy* allows the ophthalmologist to see the angle structures of the eye. Because of overlying sclera, and the way in which light is internally reflected in the eye, the angle structures cannot normally be seen unless a special contact lens, microscope, and light source are used.[15] The different zones can be differentiated by their different amounts of pigment: the corneal zone has no pigment; the trabecular meshwork catches loose iris pigment; Schlemm's canal may be seen if blood is refluxed back into the canal; and, finally, the ciliary body band is an innately pigmented structure.

Gonioscopy is primarily used to evaluate a patient who has glaucoma. It allows the ophthalmologist to decide whether the glaucoma is of the *open-, narrow-,* or *closed-angle* type. In a secondary role, it allows him to record subtle pathologic defects in the angle, which may give him a clue as to the origin of the glaucoma.

Keratometry (Ophthalmometry)[16]

The keratometer, or ophthalmometer, measures the curvature of the cornea. At first glance, the task of accurately determining the radius of curvature of a structure as tiny and as sensitive as the cornea seems formidable. In 1619, however, Father Cristoph Scheiner realized that the normal glistening cornea acts very much like a convex mirror. Therefore, he made a series of glass marbles, each of a different radius of curvature. In examining a patient, Father Scheiner had his subject stare at the open window. The size of the reflection of the window frame varied directly with the radius of curvature of the cornea. To approximate the corneal curvature, Father Scheiner compared the size of the corneal reflection with the reflections in his series of calibrated marbles. In 1796 Everard Home, son-in-law of anatomist John Hunter, and Jessie Ramsden, inventor of the Ramsden eyepiece, developed a keratometer in an attempt to prove their theory that changes in the corneal curvature are responsible for accommodation.[17] The instrument worked, although the theory did not.

It was Helmholtz, again, who made the keratometer more precise by modifying a technique, called double-image micrometry, that the astronomers were using. Instead of using the windowframe as his illuminated target, he placed an illuminated, striped target right into his machine. Because of the astronomical origin of the device, the targets were called mires, from the French astronomical term meaning meridian mark. Helmholtz's device was probably too complicated for clinical use, and so Javal and Schiotz, in 1887, used the principles of their forebears to develop a machine that focused a brightly lit target onto the cornea, measured the size of the image, and finally computed the radius of curvature all in a few simple steps (Fig. 2-21.)

The keratometer is helpful in producing a spectacles prescription for a patient with astigmatism. Nevertheless, with all the sophisticated methods of measuring refractive errors currently available, the keratometer manufacturers would have been forced out of business if not for the invention of contact lenses. To select a properly fitting corneal contact lens, we must know the curvature of the cornea. The keratometer is therefore the key instrument in the contact-lens fitter's armamentarium.

Fluorescent Staining

Fluorescein, a green dye, has been known for over 100 years. It is valuable in diagnosing eye disease because (1) it is nontoxic (it can be injected intravenously without problems), (2) it is soluble in water, blood and connective tissue, and (3) it fluoresces bright yellow-green when illuminated with blue or ultraviolet light.[18] If an abrasion of the cornea is present, applying a sterile fluorescein solution and directing a blue light on the

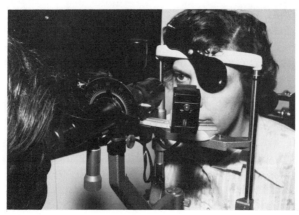

Figure 2-21. The keratometer (note the reflection of mire on the subject's cornea).

cornea will cause the abrasion to fluoresce a bright yellow-green. Once the surface epithelial cells are scraped off the cornea, laying bare the underlying stromal connective tissue, fluorescein dye is absorbed by the water of the connective tissue and glows when blue light strikes it.

Ophthalmodynamometry

The internal carotid arteries of the neck are major blood-supply routes for the brain, and occlusion of one or both of the internal carotid arteries is responsible for about one-third of the strokes in the United States.[19] It would be helpful if one could accurately measure the blood supply through the internal carotid arteries in a noninvasive way. Fortunately, the ophthalmic artery is the first branch of the internal carotid, and it gives rise to the retinal artery. This latter vessel can actually be seen with the ophthalmoscope. One can estimate the pressure in the internal carotid from the pressure in the accessible retinal artery.

Baillart, in 1912, devised an ophthalmodynamometer (ODN) to measure the pressure in the latter artery. The instrument is basically a spring gauge that indents the side of the eye while the examiner observes the retinal artery. As the indentation raises the intraocular pressure, a level is reached at which the artery starts to pulsate. At this point the interocular pressure counterbalances the systemic *diastolic* pressure, and the pulsation reflects the *systolic* breakthrough. As more pressure is applied, a level is reached at which the artery will cease pulsating. This is the *systolic* level.

In interpreting the diastolic and systolic values for each eye, the absolute values recorded are less helpful than comparing the values of one eye to the other. A difference of 15% in the pressure readings between the eyes strongly suggests an internal carotid occlusion or stenosis on the side of the low reading. In healthy, nonarteriosclerotic patients, the ophthalmic artery pressures are about 85% of the systemic blood pressure readings.[20]

Unfortunately, the test shows a significant difference between both eyes only when about 85% of an internal carotid is occluded. Lesser occlusions are masked by the collateral circulation from the other side, which helps to maintain symmetric retinal-artery pressures.

References

1. Ellis PP, Smith DL: *Handbook of Ocular Therapeutics and Pharmacology.* St. Louis, Mosby, 1973, p 11

2. Snyder C: *Our Ophthalmic Heritage.* Boston, Little Brown, 1961, p 97

3. Duke-Elder S: *System of Ophthalmology,* Vol VII. *The Foundations of Ophthalmology.* St. Louis, Mosby, 1962, p 376

4. Duke-Elder: p 394

5. Snyder: p 74

6. Mann I: *Culture, Race, Climate and Eye Disease.* Springfield, Ill, Thomas, 1966, p 13

7. Helve J: A comparative study of several diagnostic tests of color vision. Acta Ophthalmol [Suppl] 115:5, 1972

8. Taylor WOG: Practical problems of defective colour vision. Practitioner 214:654, 1975

9. Rucker CW: *A History of the Ophthalmoscope.* Rochester, Minnesota, Whiting Printers and Stationers, 1971, p 57

10. Rucker: p 13

11. Schepens CL: A new ophthalmoscope demonstration. Trans Am Acad Ophthalmol Otolaryngol 51:298, 1947

12. Duke-Elder: pp 337–355

13. Hertel E: Ein einfaches Exophthalmometer. Arch Ophthalmol 60: 171, 1905

14. Duane TD: *Clinical Ophthalmology,* Vol 2. Hagerstown, Maryland, Harper & Row, 1978, p 15

15. Duke-Elder: p 270

16. Southall JPC: *Mirrors, Prisms and Lenses.* New York, Macmillan, 1933, p 698

17. Levene JR: Early studies in visual optics, with particular reference to the mechanism of accommodation. Proc Royal Microbiol Soc 2:139, 1967

18. Lebensohn JE: Fluorescein in ophthalmology. Am J Ophthalmol 67:442, 1969

19. Marshall J: The management of occlusion and stenosis of the internal carotid artery. Neurology (Minneap) 16:1087, 1966

20. Hayreh SS: The ophthalmic artery. In: *Vision and Circulation*. Edited by JS Cant. St. Louis, Mosby, 1976, pp 171–179

Chapter 3

Blindness

Almost half a million Americans are legally blind, and each year 30,000 more Americans lose their sight. The estimated annual cost to public welfare agencies for services to the blind is over a half-billion dollars.[1] To the ophthalmologist, these statistics represent a failure of modern medicine and illustrate the need for continued research on eye diseases.

Legally, corrected vision of 20/200 or worse or a visual field of 20% or less, in the better eye, constitutes blindness. A person with 20/200 vision can recognize other people and objects, and most legally blind people can see to some extent; 75% see about 20/200, 12% see only light and dark, and 12% see nothing.

Causes

That 68% of the blind population is over 65 years of age may indicate that aging is the major cause of blindness. More specifically, however, the major causes of blindness, in decreasing order of frequency, are retinal and choroidal disease, cataract, glaucoma, optic nerve atrophy, corneal disease, and prenatal disease (Table 3-1).[1]

Retinal Disease

The leading cause of blindness is retinal disease. This category accounts for 75% of all blindness and includes such conditions as *senile macular degeneration, diabetic retinopathy, hypertensive retinopathy,* and *retinitis pigmentosa.*

Table 3-1. Causes of New Blindness[a,1]

Cause	Percentage
Retinal and choroidal disease (diabetic retinopathy, senile macular degeneration)	46
Cataract	17
Glaucoma	14
Optic nerve atrophy	6
Corneal disease	3
Other (e.g., congenital disease, trauma)	9
Not reported	5

[a]Data current on June 30, 1974.

Cataracts

A *cataract* is a progressive opacity of the lens, not very incapacitating in its early stages, but leading to debilitating blindness if left untreated. Many cataract victims have such fear of the treatment, i.e., surgical removal, that they prefer to live with the disease rather than undergo the operation. Almost 500,000 cataract operations are performed in the United States each year, 95% of them successful; still, some three million Americans have debilitating cataracts.

Very preliminary experiments in our laboratory on a filter that would allow the eye to see through cataract tissue[2] occasioned a demonstration of the fears and hopes of cataract victims. Although the filter we were developing showed little promise of ever being useful in humans, hundreds of elderly people wrote to us describing their fear of surgery and offering themselves as experimental subjects for the development of the filter. We, of course, had to tell each one that the experiments were only in the earliest stages and that we recommended surgery as their best chance for sight restoration.

Glaucoma

Glaucoma refers to a group of eye diseases characterized by increased intraocular pressure that eventually results in damage to the optic nerve, which ultimately leads to blindness. When glaucoma does result in blindness, it is termed *endstage,* or *absolute, glaucoma.* Endstage glaucoma is the second leading cause of blindness in this country, afflicting some 14% of all blind people. Glaucoma claims eight times as many nonwhite victims as it does white,[3] a fact that may simply reflect the differing availability of eye care and education to these populations. Whatever the reason, glaucoma-caused blindness is especially tragic because, with early diagnosis and treatment of glaucoma, blindness need never occur. In fact, 800,000 Americans are presently under treatment for the disease. If they diligently follow the treatment prescribed by their doctors, few, if any, should ever lose their sight.

Optic-Nerve Atrophy

Nine percent of all blindness is due to *atrophy of the optic nerve*. Such atrophy may be caused by a total interruption in the blood supply to the nerve, which might occur in arteriosclerosis of the ophthalmic artery, giant cell arteritis of the ophthalmic artery, or occlusion of the central retinal artery. The neuronal elements of the optic nerve may be destroyed in optic neuritis, chronic papilledema, or tumor invasion of the nerve.

Corneal Disease

Corneal disease, which accounts for 3% of all blindness in the United States, includes all the infections and inherited conditions that cause the cornea to turn a lifeless gray or white. However, this figure of 3% does represent a triumph of American medicine in one respect. In most less-developed countries, corneal disease resulting from malnutrition, trachoma (a chlamydial infection), and untreated bacterial infections is the leading cause of blindness. Public health measures and education are the strongest weapons for controlling these serious corneal conditions.

Prenatal Disease

Finally, *prenatal disease,* a vast collection of inherited or congenital diseases, accounts for the remainder of the causes of blindness. Here again, we can thank a small group of medical researchers for materially decreasing the size of this group. In 1941, for example, Dr. Norman McAllister Gregg noted a surprisingly high incidence of congenital cataracts after a rubella outbreak. By carefully questioning the mothers, he discovered that 68 of the 70 mothers with afflicted children recalled having a viral infection during pregnancy. Ultimately, scientists discovered the rubella virus living in the congenital cataracts of these children, and now, with vaccination against this form of measles, we can prevent cataracts due to maternal rubella infection.

Immunosuppressive Agents

Another small but significant recent cause of blindness is related to the immunosuppressive agents now used to treat certain forms of cancer or to help transplanted organs survive. Unfortunately, these powerful agents impair the body's normal defenses. Thus, blinding ocular infections are now reported in these patients from such opportunistic organisms as the cytomegalovirus, the herpes zoster and herpes simplex viruses, and by such fungi as *Candida, Aspergillus, Mucor,* and *Cryptococcus.*[4]

Hope for the Blind

In 1940 the incidence of blindness was 175 people per 100,000 population.[5] Now it is a little less. Does this mean that we have made little progress in prevention and treatment of blindness since then? Definitely not! Recall that 68% of all our blind are 65 years of age or older. Learning how to extend the lives of our citizens has resulted in increased incidence of many debilitating, degenerative diseases, some of which lead to blindness. Even so, the overall incidence of blindness has decreased somewhat.

After World War II, the widespread use of antibiotics reversed the ravages of trachoma, gonorrheal ophthalmia, and other corneal infections. Introduction of corticosteroids in the early 1950s[6] controlled the blinding effects of iritis and significantly reduced immune rejection of corneal transplants. Widespread education encouraged the public to have glaucoma checks in their 50s and 60s, thus isolating glaucoma and arresting its progress at early stages. Enforced use of protective goggles eliminated many of the industrial injuries that lead to blindness. Since the 1950s, the equipment for cataract surgery has steadily improved, increasing the operation's success rate. The 1970s saw the initiation of a successful campaign against diabetic retinopathy. Laser treatment has been an encouraging start. By 1974 the techniques of vitrectomy brought sight to about one-third of the diabetics who had been blinded by hemorrhage into the vitreous. These techniques allow the surgeon to carefully remove the bloodstained vitreous without damaging the retina, and to replace it with a clear substitute such as isotonic saline.

Although the pace at which cure or prevention of blindness has progressed in the past 30 years has been breathtaking, the most difficult causes of blindness remain unremedied. Many of these conditions are closely related to the aging process itself, and so their cures become that much more challenging.

The greatest hope of conquering eye disease probably lies in allowing research scientists the luxury of keeping open minds, unbound by the dogmas that our "experts" so confidently establish. At the Bowman lecture of 1888, the famous pioneer of corneal surgery, Henry Power, explained how nearly all eye diseases were simply the sequel to sexual indulgence.[7] Just think where we would be had everyone followed Dr. Power's philosophy.

Braille

Louis Braille was accidentally blinded as a child. After completing his education at the National Institute for the Blind in Paris in 1819, he stayed on as a teacher. By 1834 he had developed a system of 63 combinations of 6 raised, palpable dots to represent the letters of the alphabet, certain common words, frequent letter combinations, and musical terms. ("W" was missing from Braille's original system because the French alphabet contains no "W.") By 1865 an American named Joel Smith invented a mechanical Braille writer, a device which embossed the desired combination of dots on a flat piece of paper lying on a hand slate. Ultimately, the typewriter principle was applied to Braille, and in 1892 the Hall Braille writer was introduced, opening the way for the mass printing of books in Braille.[5]

Guide Dogs

The use of guide dogs for the blind was started in Austria in 1819 by Johann Wilhelm Klein. Since the inception of the program in the United States in 1929, 4,000 blind people have been successfully trained to use dogs.[5] It has been estimated that only 1 blind person in 100 benefits from using a dog,[1] because most blind people have far too much sight to rely on the guide dog and others who lose their sight after age 60 (the bulk of the blind population) find the training course too taxing, both physically and mentally. By and large, the guide dog is useful only to the young, sightless person.

The White Cane

A tall staff has helped the blind to avoid obstacles since ancient times. During World War II, however, the design and use of the cane was significantly improved by Dr. Richard E. Hoover at the Army's center for the war-blinded in Valley Forge, Pennsylvania.[5] The cane was lengthened to give a scanning range of 5 feet, and its design was altered to integrate its swing with natural body movement. The cane is white to signify that the user is blind.

Electronic Devices

The most promising recent development in aids for the blind is a reading machine that acts much like a miniature TV camera moving across the printed page.[8] This device has 144 tiny light-receptors that identify each letter or numeral below it and transmit the information to one of 144 corresponding vibrating points located on a small plate worn on the blind

Table 3-2. Agencies Concerned with the Blind[a]

Boston Aid to the Blind, Inc.
Boston Center for Blind Children
Blind Leadership Club of Boston
Massachusetts Commission for the Blind
Massachusetts Association for the Blind
Carroll Rehabilitation Center for the Blind
Catholic Charitable Bureau of the Archdiocese of Boston
Protestant Guild for the Blind, Inc.
Jewish Family Services
Lighthouse, New York City

[a]Only Boston and Massachusetts agencies are listed, but they are typical of those found in every major United States city.

reader's index finger. The blind person learns to understand the code of vibrations sensed by his finger. Some trained subjects can read up to 60 words per minute with this device.

The engineering division of the American Foundation for the Blind has recently developed a Braille electronic calculator that performs percentages and the four major arithmetic functions.

Role of the Physician

Generally, the ophthalmologist is the first doctor to confirm the diagnosis of blindness, and so it is his responsibility to set the blind patient on a path that will allow the patient to lead an active life. The blind patient will face economic, emotional, and travel problems. Over the years, agencies and experts have developed ways of helping the blind person in these areas, and the physician or nurse dealing with a blind person has the responsibility of helping him to contact the appropriate local agency. Table 3-2 lists the agencies typically found in most geographic areas.

References

1. *Vision Research Program Planning,* Vol 1 [DHEW No. (NIH) 75-654]. Washington, DC, U.S. Government Printing Office, 1974, pp 1-4

2. Miller D, Zuckerman JL, Reynolds GO: Holographic filter to negate the effect of cataract. Arch Ophthalmol 90:323, 1973

3. Hiller R, Kohn HA: Blindness from glaucoma. Am J Ophthalmol 80:62, 1975

4. Cogan DG: Immunosuppression and eye disease. Am J Ophthalmol 83:777, 1977

5. Chevigny H, Braverman S: *The Adjustment of the Blind.* New Haven, Yale University Press, 1950, pp 89–116

6. Hench PS, Kendall EC, Slocumb CH, et al: The effect of a hormone of the adrenal cortex (17-hydroxy-11-dehydrocorticosterone, compound E) and of pituitary adrenocorticotropic hormone on rheumatoid arthritis. Proc Staff Meet Mayo Clin 24:181, 1949

7. Trevor-Roper PD (ed.): *Recent Advances in Ophthalmology.* Edinburgh, Churchill Livingstone, 1975, p 308

8. Bliss J: A reading machine with tactile display. In: *Visual Prosthesis, The Interdisciplinary Dialogue.* Edited by TD Sterling, EA Bering Jr, SV Pollack, et al. New York, Academic Press, 1971, p 259

Chapter 4

Eye Exercises

In 1942 Aldous Huxley told the world that seeing was an art that could be learned. In his book *The Art of Seeing,* Huxley told how he had suffered as a teenager from a devastating inflammation of both corneas that ultimately resulted in dense scarring, vision of 20/400 in one eye, and only light-dark perception in the other eye. In 1939, while in California, he learned of Mrs. Margaret D. Corbett and her method of visual reeducation. Following her instructions, the corneal opacities began to clear, and within two years, at age 45, he could read effortlessly without his glasses.[1] In essence, the book strongly suggested that if ophthalmologists stop using such mechanical palliative devices as glasses and concentrate instead on reeducation, the damaged eye would also heal.

The idea of treating refractive errors and eye pathology with exercises seems to have been popularized in earnest in 1920 by an ophthalmologist, Dr. William Horatio Bates. In his book *The Cure of Imperfect Sight By Treatment Without Glasses,* Bates claimed that such deformations of the eye as those which occur in myopia, presbyopia, and astigmatism were due to abnormal strain of the extraocular muscles. The cure, then, was accomplished by relaxation through concentration. In "resting," for example, one closed his eyes and thought of agreeable things; in "palming" one covered his eyes with his palms and concentrated on seeing black; and in the "Big Swing" one stood erect and twisted both torso and head from side to side, allowing the eyes to move freely with the swing. With each exercise session, one was always to practice reading an eye-test card, and was advised to study it continually, striving to read the smallest type.

There are still some who feel that the vested interests of the health-care establishments are served by using such unnatural modalities as spectacles, surgery, and medicines when less expensive methods of exercise and natural foods can achieve the same ends. The scientific claims of the Huxley-Bates method were set to rest in a study of 103 myopes who were given the Bates training and then assessed by a panel of ophthalmologists and optometrists. With the possible exception that some patients learned to interpret blurred images more carefully, and that others thought they could see better even though there was no actual improvement, the study showed no effect of visual training in the treatment of myopia.

Could Huxley actually read without glasses after mastering the Bates therapeutic course? In an article that appeared in the *Saturday Review*, Bennett Cerf related an episode about Huxley that seemed to set the record straight. Huxley was reading a prepared address to a Hollywood gathering, most of whom had heard of his miraculous cure, and Cerf noted the following:

When he arose to make his address, he wore no glasses, and evidently experienced no difficulty in reading the paper he had planted on the lectern. Had the exercises really given him normal vision? I, along with twelve hundred other guests watched in astonishment while he rattled glibly on. Then suddenly, he faltered and the disturbing truth became obvious. He wasn't reading his address at all. He had learned it by heart. To refresh his memory, he brought the paper closer and closer to his eyes. When it was only an inch or so away, he still couldn't read it, and had to fish for a magnifying glass in his pocket to make the typing visible to him. It was an agonizing moment.[2]

Poor Readers

Not too long ago, a well-known TV newscaster came to our office for a routine eye examination. During the exam, the reading card was mistakenly handed to him upside down. He smiled and rapidly read through the entire card. "My father and uncle can also read upside down. I guess reading skills are inherited," he concluded.

One family story does not prove very much, but there have been larger studies. In one, Hermann evaluated 45 sets of twins, of whom at least one twin of each set had a reading disability.[3] Of the 12 pairs of identical monozygotic twins, both twins of all 12 pairs showed the identical disability. Of the 33 sets of nonidentical (dizygotic) twins, both twins of 11 pairs, or 33%, had identical reading problems. These figures help support the conclusion of the TV newscaster.

It appears that the potential for exceptional reading skills as well as for deficient reading skills are basically inherited. If this is true, then reading disabilities, like inborn errors of metabolism, are never outgrown. This last conclusion is supported by the work of Margaret Rawson, who followed patients with dyslexia for 20 years. She found that, although the educational attainments of these people were no less than those of normal readers, many continued to find reading and spelling embarrassing tasks.[4]

Before we get too deeply into this section, it might be appropriate to ask why a book about eyes and eye disease deals with reading disabilities when reading is really the province of educators and teachers. There are some eye-care professionals who feel that reading-disability problems relate to refractive errors, eye movements, eye-muscle balance, and difficulty in differentiating right from left. On this basis, training courses, often lasting for years, are offered to children who are poor readers. Time is spent following a rolling marble around a pizza pan, balancing on a board, drilling on the trampoline, and performing exercises in which both eyes are trained to work together. Is there any evidence that eye defects, or ocular muscle imbalance, produce reading disability? On the contrary, numerous studies have demonstrated repeatedly that the presence of eye defects and ocular-muscle imbalance has little or nothing to do with reading ability.[5-7]

Why, then, does a sophisticated public support such training programs? The United States today is a credential society: degrees from colleges and postgraduate institutions are the credentials needed to achieve success, and these credentials will not be available to any student with poor reading skills. Thus, to the concerned parent of a poor reader, it makes sense to hear that the child is a poor reader because he did not learn to use his eyes, hands, body, and perceptual parts of the brain in the proper natural sequence. The exercises are an attempt to go back to square one and relearn the necessary skills of perception in the proper order. With over 20% of our school population classified as reading failures, it is not surprising that parents and well-meaning eye practitioners will try anything that seems logical and natural.

Unfortunately, these modern methods of reeducating cognitive skills through eye-body exercises do not have a convincing record in reading improvements.[8] Can reading skills be improved, then, or are poor readers doomed from kindergarten? Most school systems have programs for poor readers. The aim of such training is to bring the letter, or word, into the interpretive centers of the brain through the other sensory channels. Letters are traced by the fingers, or auditory associations are made. Slowly, the alphabet is blended into words and phrases. Children trained this way are rarely avid readers, but they are able to function at a higher level than previously.

Dyslexia

Dyslexia is the term used to describe an affliction of children who read significantly below their mental ages or who, in other words, are very poor readers. The typical dyslexic child is male and left-handed, reverses letters (confuses *p* for *q*, or *u* for *n*, or *stop* for *pots*), finds it hard to pronounce strange words, has a normal or superior IQ, is better than average in arithmetic, and may have emotional problems.[9] It is still not clear whether poor reading performance produces emotional problems, or whether emotional problems interfere with learning to read. Happily, dyslexics need not be social or professional failures. History's list of successful dyslexics includes Winston Churchill, Harvey Cushing, Thomas Edison, Albert Einstein, Woodrow Wilson, and John Hunter.

Speed Reading

It was often said that former President Kennedy could read at least 1500 words per minute, while the average adult reads 250 words per minute. Although the intellect of the average American adult cannot be retrained to function at President Kennedy's level, reading speed can certainly be improved. To understand how this can be achieved, it will be helpful first to review the durations of physiologic events that take place during the act of reading.[10]

A visual acuity of 20/60 is required to see ordinary print at the usual reading distance. Studies indicate that such an acuity is attainable with a 5° field surrounding the fovea. At the usual reading distance of 33 cm, a 5° field includes 3 average-sized words. The speed of light is such that we can assume a three-word phrase to be focused onto the retina instantly. The conduction time from eye to brain is 0.1 second, and processing requires another 0.1 second. It then takes 0.05 second to move the eyes to the next phrase. Therefore, if reading three words takes about 0.25 of a second, the maximum reading speed attainable is between 720 and 800 words per minute.[10] To achieve speeds of 1500 words per minute, the reader must skim, i.e., arbitrarily skip words and phrases. Skimming is effective when combined with a preliminary review of the table of contents, summary paragraphs, headings, and the like. The actual skimming fills the details into the conceptual framework achieved by the survey.

Speed-reading courses teach the student first to survey the material, and then to convert from oral to visual reading by driving the student to pick up 2 or 3 words per fixation and by forcing his eyes to stay one step ahead of a pacing device. Controlled studies have shown that speed reading courses are effective for reading fiction and newspaper text, but less effective for scientific and technical works.[11]

Orthoptics

Orthoptics is a science that deals with training the individual to use both eyes together to attain comfortable binocular vision. It is primarily concerned with patients suffering from *strabismus* and *amblyopia*.

Strabismus is a term that means crossed eyes or walleyes *(exotropia)*. A patient with strabismus is said to have *fusion* if he has the brain capability of coordinating and fusing together the impulses received from each eye. Pre- and postoperative orthoptic exercises in strabismic patients with fusion often help to maintain a straight-eyed position and allow the patient to enjoy a richer visual experience.

Amblyopia is a condition of reduced vision that is not caused by either organic disease or errors of refraction. In a strabismic patient, amblyopia occurs primarily in the eye that turns inward or outward. The essential element in amblyopia treatment is to force the weak eye to develop vision while the good eye is covered. This is usually achieved by patching the good eye and training the weak eye to see finer and finer details.

Orthoptic exercises can also be helpful in patients who complain of eye fatigue. In these patients, reinforcing stronger eye-convergence patterns with special orthoptic exercises often results in a decrease in the complaint of eye strain.

References

1. Snyder C: Bates, Huxley and myself. Int Ophthalmol Clin 2:921, 1962

2. Quoted in Pollack P: *The Truth About Eye Exercises.* New York, Chilton, 1956, p 7

3. Hermann K: *Reading Disability: A Medical Study of Word Blindness and Related Handicaps.* Springfield, Ill, Thomas, 1959, pp 28–84

4. Rawson MD: *Developmental Language Disability: Adult Accomplishments of Dyslexic Boys.* Baltimore, Johns Hopkins Press, 1968, p 24

5. Bettman JW Jr, Stern EL, Whitsell LJ, et al: Cerebral dominancy in developmental dyslexia: role of the ophthalmologist. Arch Ophthalmol 78:722, 1967

6. Norn MS, Rindziunski E, Skydsgaard H: Ophthalmologic and orthoptic examination in dyslexics. Acta Ophthalmol (Kbh) 47:147, 1969

7. Goldberg HK, Guthrie JT: Evaluation of visual perceptual factors in reading disability. J Pediatr Ophthalmol 9:18, 1972

8. Carlson V, Greenspoon K: The uses and abuses of visual training for children with perceptual motor learning problems. Am J Optom 45:161, 1968

9. Goldberg HK, Schiffman GB: *Dyslexia, Problems of Reading Disabilities,* New York, Grune & Stratton, 1972, p 145

10. Miller D: A review of speed reading theory and techniques for the ophthalmologist. Am J Ophthalmol 62:334, 1966

11. desIslets JCM: An investigation of the use of accelerated reading skills at the USAF Academy, Fall 1961–62. In: *Speed Reading: Practice and Procedures.* Edited by RD Stauffer. School of Education, University of Delaware, 1963

Chapter 5

Refractive Errors

Ninety million Americans—almost one-half of the population—wear glasses. It seems odd that the eye, such a sophisticated and ingenious organ, should be, for half of us, often out of focus.[1] It might be useful to look into the focusing elements of the eye and see how they develop.

Normal Eye Function

Lenses

To understand how the eye focuses, one must understand how a lens works. Lenses are graded in *diopters* (D). The diopter is an arbitrary quantity obtained by dividing 100 by the *focal length,* in centimeters, of a lens. The *focal length* of a lens is the distance from the optical center of that lens to its *focal point,* the point where parallel light rays are converged by that lens. (For example, a lens with a focal length of 5 cm is a 20 D lens: $100 \div 5 = 20$.) Lenses with short focal lengths are said to be strong lenses; those with long focal lengths, weak lenses.

Obviously, not all lenses converge light rays; there are lenses that diverge light rays. Converging lenses are referred to as *plus lenses* (Fig. 5-1). The lens in the preceding paragraph would be listed as a +20 D lens. Diverging lenses are referred to as *minus lenses.* Describing a diverging lens requires an example. Imagine that parallel light rays enter the left side of a lens and are diverged as they emerge from the right side of the lens. The diverging rays appear to emanate from a point on the left side of the lens (Fig. 5-2)—a "negative" focus. The distance between that point and the center of that lens is the "negative" focal length. Accordingly, a

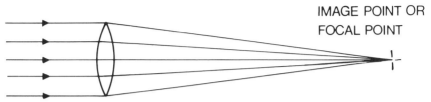

IMAGE POINT OR
FOCAL POINT

Figure 5-1. Plus lens. Parallel rays converge to a focal point. (Artist: Laurel Cook.)

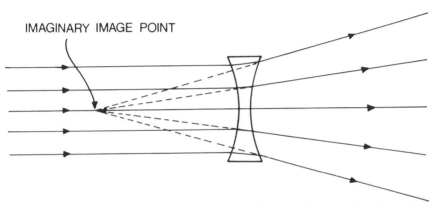

IMAGINARY IMAGE POINT

Figure 5-2. Minus lens. Parallel rays diverge, as if emanating from the focal point. (Artist: Laurel Cook.)

diverging lens with a "negative" focal length of 5 cm would be a -20 D lens $(100 \div [-5] = -20)$.

Emmetropization

When the cornea, lens, and eye length are perfectly coordinated (i.e., when parallel rays entering the eye come to a focus on the retina), the eye is called *emmetropic*. As will be discussed in subsequent paragraphs, if the rays focus in front of the retina, the eye is said to be *myopic;* and if the rays converge beyond the retina, the eye is said to be *hyperopic.*

Any optical system must be precise, and the eye is no exception. Consider an imaginary emmetropic eye, filled primarily with physiologic fluid (with a given index of refraction), and with a cornea and lens whose combined optical power is 60 D. According to a complicated formula, the retina will be 2.4 cm behind the anterior surface of the cornea. If we are able to increase this corneal-retinal distance to 2.5 cm (for the sake of observation), and if all other conditions remain constant, this eye will now be more than 2 D myopic and would barely be able to read the 20/200 letter at the top of a Snellen chart.

Within the constraints of such precision, it is an extraordinary fact that most eyes appear to stay close to the emmetropic state through infancy and childhood, in spite of a significant enlargement of the eyeball itself.[2] The average neonatal eye is 1.9 cm from cornea to retina. The average adult eye is 2.4 cm in length. Such a 0.5-cm increase in axial length should lead to the development of about 15 D of myopia. Just to place things in perspective, a 15-D myope wears lenses thick enough to truly distort the appearance of his face and eyes. Yet, by age 3, the average eye almost reaches adult dimensions, and actually has about 2 D of hyperopia. This tendency toward emmetropization is accomplished primarily by a change in the shape of the lens of the eye. As it enlarges, the lens slowly converts from an almost spherical shape to a flatter form with less refractive power. It seems that the genes of each individual are programmed with a coordinated pattern of growth for axial length and lens shape. Unfortunately, this amazing process of emmetropization is not perfect—as evidenced by the many Americans who wear glasses.

What are the limits of the process of emmetropization? Seventy-five percent of the population has 0 D–2 D of hyperopia. Because in most people under 40 years of age 2 D of hyperopia can be compensated by the accommodation of the eye lens, these people need not wear glasses. Hyperopia of +2 D to +6 D appears in 10% of the population, and myopia between 0 D and −4 D appears in another 10% of the population. It is these last 2 groups who need glasses, plus most people over 45 years of age, who need reading glasses to compensate for diminishing powers of accommodation. Let us focus more closely on the people who wear most of the spectacles in America, those with *ametropia* (as opposed to emmetropia), i.e., those with defective coordination of the refractive elements of the eyes.

Ametropia

Myopia

In *myopia* (nearsightedness), parallel rays entering the eye come to a focus in front of the retina, which thereby receives a blurred image (Fig. 5-3). Myopia may stem from an eye whose cornea and/or lens possess refractive power that is too great for its focal length, or from an eye that is too long for the refractive power of its cornea and lens. The proper minus lens in front of that eye could cause parallel rays of light to diverge just enough to focus on the retina.

Myopia is certainly the more inconvenient of the refractive errors. For these patients, the world is a perpetual blur, and they see clearly only those things that are close to their eyes. Before they are fitted with glasses, most myopes learn to close their eyes so that only a thin crack is left open. Through such a slit, they see more clearly as they achieve somewhat the effect of a lensless pinhole camera.

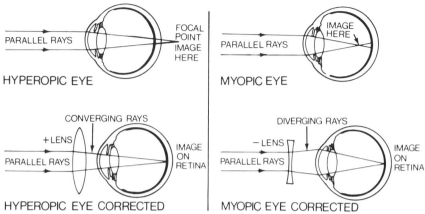

Figure 5-3. *Top left:* Hyperopic eye focuses parallel rays behind the retina. *Lower left:* Proper plus lens focuses parallel rays onto the retina. *Top right:* Myopic eye focuses parallel rays into the vitreous. *Lower right:* Proper minus lens refocuses parallel rays onto the retina. (Courtesy of American Optical Corporation.)

Myopes may be divided into two categories. The high myopes, those with over 4 D, include about 1% of the population. In general, eyes of over 4 D of myopia have a greater axial length. The chances for retinal detachment increase as the eye elongates and the choroid and retina are stretched and thinned.

The other category, comprising the bulk of the myopic population, has errors from ¼ D to 4 D. These patients usually have a genetic predisposition to myopia, which appears to be elicited by heavy use of the eyes for reading. A study of the refractive status of an isolated, genetically pure Eskimo village in Pt. Barrow, Alaska, for instance, revealed that while there was almost no myopia in the parents and grandparents, the incidence of myopia was about 60% in those under 25 years of age. The young population had been taught to read; the older group read very little.[3] Other studies in the United States have shown that about 10% of grade-school children, 20% of high-school population, 40% of the college population, and 50% of graduate students are myopic.[4,5] This latter group of people in their twenties has a much higher incidence of myopia than has a comparable age grouping who do not go to graduate school. Thus it seems that there is a gene for mild myopia, which expresses itself if the subject reads a great deal during his teens and twenties.

Hyperopia

Hyperopia (farsightedness) is the direct opposite of myopia. Here parallel light rays are intercepted by the retina before they come to a focus. The farsighted eye either is shorter than the normal eye or has refractive power too weak for the length of the eye. In either case, the rays from an object will never focus on the retina (Fig. 5-3).

Often the hyperopic eye can adjust itself to clear vision through accommodation. The blurring of the image indirectly causes the ciliary body to contract, increasing the refractive power of the lens. This added optical power may sometimes be sufficient to compensate for the hyperopia so that the rays will focus on the retina. With increasing age, however, the lens of the eye slowly loses its ability to accommodate. Thus, the hyperope often must use spectacles with plus lenses, which supply enough extra converging power to focus the world on his retina.

The hyperope, when young, rarely needs glasses. In addition to the accommodation response, there is a reflex known as the *near reflex*, which automatically forces both eyes to converge when the eye accommodates. The reflex appears to have a logical basis since we usually accommodate to examine an object at close range, and we usually converge our eyes onto the object at the same time. Unfortunately, over 2% of the child population has *strabismus*, a condition in which the eye turns in or out. In most cases one eye turns inward *(esotropia)*. Of the esotropic group, about one in ten can straighten the eye if the hyperopia is corrected with glasses, so overaccommodation is not necessary to compensate for the hyperopia. Thus, measurement for hyperopia is important in the patient with esotropia.

Astigmatism

Another type of refractive error, known as *astigmatism,* results from an abnormally shaped cornea. The normal cornea is uniform and spherical, somewhat like a rounded soup spoon, while the curvature of the astigmatic cornea is not uniform in all meridians, but is much like an elongated soup spoon (Fig. 5-4). Therefore, the refractive power of the astigmatic cornea is not uniform in all meridians. A ray of parallel light can never be focused to a single point by an astigmatic cornea; an uncorrected astigmat will look at a spot of light and proclaim that it looks like an ellipse. The direction of the line (the major axis of the ellipse) is the direction of the corneal astigmatism. A line perpendicular to the meridian of the astigmatism is called the axis of astigmatism.

The development of the keratometer has allowed us to learn a great deal about astigmatism. The keratometer divides the frontal plane of the cornea into a circle of 360° and can measure the refracting power in any of 360 meridians. In a spherical cornea, the refracting power will be the same in every meridian. In the astigmat, there is a meridian which has the greatest refracting power, and another meridian 90° away where the refracting power is the least. The latter meridian is known as the axis of the astigmatism.

Astigmatism can be present by itself, or in combination with hyperopia or myopia. A person with astigmatism does not simply see the world

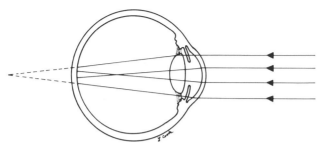

Figure 5-4. Astigmatism. Two sets of rays focus in front of and behind the retina. (Artist: Laurel Cook.)

as a blur, but as a distorted blur. If the axis of astigmatism is horizontal (i.e., 180°), everyone looks tall and thin. Astigmatism is corrected by a cylindrical lens, an optical device with focusing power in only one meridian.

Presbyopia

Presbyopia, the loss of ability to focus sharply on objects close to the eye, develops as one reaches middle age. At age 10, a child with normal vision can focus clearly upon insects and rock details as near to his eyes as the tip of his nose. He probably can accommodate 15 D. By age 45 our accommodation is only about 2 or 3 D, which means we have to hold our books and magazines 30 to 50 cm away; and at age 65, the lens in our eye has lost just about all of its elasticity and accommodative power.

Middle-aged patients, accordingly, must wear reading glasses that provide added focusing power and help to focus details at close range. Reading glasses help to extend our productive lives—can you imagine a modern society in which middle-aged scholars, craftsmen, executives, and doctors could not study or read print unless they were myopic? Unfortunately, only what is close to the eyes appears clear with reading glasses; such glasses render us artificially myopic for distance vision. Benjamin Franklin, frustrated by this blur, invented bifocals, spectacles that are divided into two lenses per eye. Dr. Franklin's bifocals had an upper lens for distance vision and a lower half (called the *add*) for reading.

Examination and Corrrection

Refractions

Refraction is the examination performed by the ophthalmologist or optometrist to determine the strength of the glasses that a patient may need. Originally, i.e., from about 1300 until 1860, this examination consisted simply of allowing the patient to choose from a series of readymade eyeglasses. With the development of a set of calibrated and reproducible trial lenses that could be placed in a trial frame, Professor Freunmueller ushered in a more scientifically sound refraction. By 1864, Donders and Snellen had developed a series of tests that helped to determine the most accurate lens for each eye.[6]

Although our instrumentation is now more elegant and precise, the principles of refraction have changed little since the 1860s. In essence, the refractionist first determines the approximate amount and type of error by using a *retinoscope,* an *automatic refractor,* or simply the patient's old spectacles prescription. A combination of lenses equalling this approximate correction is placed before the patient's eyes. Extra lenses are then added until the examiner arrives at a combination of lens with which the patient sees the target in the sharpest manner.

Pinhole Effect

Figure 5-5 shows how a pinhole constricts a narrow bundle of out-of-focus rays, preventing them from fanning out into a large blurred circle on the retina. Can one quantitate the amount of ametropia overcome by a pinhole? As one might expect from the nature of the pinhole effect, small pinholes less than 1 mm in diameter are very effective at focusing, but induce annoying diffraction patterns and make things appear much darker. Most efficient pinholes are between 1 mm and 1.5 mm in diameter. If the target is bright enough, such a pinhole can help maintain sharp vision and compensate for about 5 D of refractive error.[7] The pinhole device has its greatest use in the examining room, differentiating the poor vision of most refractive errors from the poor vision of ocular disease.

It has been said that the nonemmetropic members of the old New York Yankees used weak concentrations of pilocarpine eyedrops to constrict their pupils in order to see more clearly on the baseball field—an example of a practical application of the pinhole effect. The pinhole effect has also been used by older patients with glaucoma who use pupil-contracting (miotic) eyedrops. These patients, too presbyopic to achieve ciliary muscle contraction, often are able to read without glasses when using these drops.

The Spectacle Prescription

Prescriptions for corrective glasses follow a straightforward system, as shown in the following examples. The abbreviations O.D. and O.S. denote *oculus dexter* and *oculus sinister,* Latin for right eye and left eye, respectively.

Example 1. The instruction

O.D. +2.00
O.S. +2.50

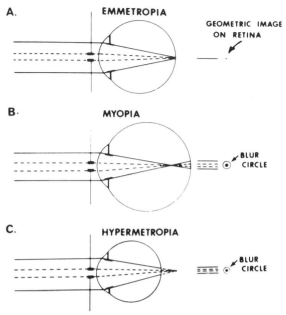

A. EMMETROPIA

GEOMETRIC IMAGE
ON RETINA

B. MYOPIA

BLUR
CIRCLE

C. HYPERMETROPIA

BLUR
CIRCLE

Figure 5-5. Principle of the pinhole effect. The effect of a pinhole introduced in front of an emmetropic eye, a myopic eye, and a hypermetropic eye, respectively (neglecting the effect of diffraction). The pinhole has no effect on the emmetropic eye **A**, but in both **B** and **C** the size of the blur-circle on the retina decreases with the pinhole aperture. (Reprinted with permission from Rubin ML: *Optics for Clinicians.* Gainesville, Fla, Triad Scientific Publications, 1974, p 187.)

means that the right eye, which is hyperopic, needs a +2.00 D lens. The left eye, also hyperopic, requires a +2.50 lens.

Example 2. The prescription

O.D. −1.75
O.S. −2.25

means that the right eye, which is myopic, requires a −1.75 D lens, i.e., the right eye is 1.75 D myopic. The left is 2.25 D myopic.

Example 3. The prescription

O.D. +2.00 = −1.75 × 180
O.S. +2.00 = −1.50 × 170

means that the right eye is 2 D hyperopic and also has 1.75 D astigmatism at axis 180°. The left eye, similarly, is 2 D hyperopic with an astigmatism of 1.5 D at axis 170°.

Example 4. The instruction

O.D. −4.75 = −.100 × 90
O.S. −4.75 = −1.00 × 90 add =2.50 O.U.

means that both eyes have 4.75 D of myopia and also 1 D of astigmatism at axis 90°. "Add =2.50" indicates that the prescription +2.50 D lens is added to the lower segment of the bifocal for both eyes (O.U.).

Table 5-1 shows how these instructions to the lens maker would appear on the doctor's prescription pad.

Headaches in Relation to Refractive Errors

Both patients and their doctors believe that errors of refraction or ocular-muscular imbalance often cause headaches. This belief dates back at least to 1876 when S. Weir Mitchell wrote: "What I desire therefore to make clear to the profession at large is that there are many headaches which are due to disorders of the refractive or accommodative apparatus of the eyes."[8]

But is this true? Dr. Malcom Cameron, an Australian ophthalmologist, set out to investigate this theory by analyzing 50 patients who were referred to him by other physicians with the complaint of headaches.[9] Of the 50 patients, 36% had headaches of a migraine nature, 54% of a nervous tension origin, and only 10% of possibly ocular origin. Dr. Cameron then took his study one step further. Since eye strain should logically lead to headaches in presbyopic patients and hyperopic patients who use excessive amounts of accommodation, he studied these groups. Of 50 presbyopic patients, only 6 (a bit over 10%) complained of headaches. Most patients simply reported that they had difficulty seeing small print. Of 15 hyperopic patients, 2 (a bit over 10%) complained of headaches when they used their eyes. We are left with evidence suggesting that refractive errors rarely cause headaches. It should be added, however, that when the headache *is* related to the refractive error, prescription of the proper pair of glasses does alleviate the headache.

Table 5-1. A Typical Corrective Lens Prescription

Eye	Sphere[a]	Cylinder[b]	Axis[c]
O.D.	–4.75	–1.00	90
O.S.	–4.75	–1.00	90
	Add = 2.50		

[a]*Sphere:* the spheric element that corrects hyperopia or myopia.
[b]*Cylinder:* the cylindric element that corrects the astigmatism.
[c]*Axis:* the orientation of the cylinder, 180° being horizontal.

Sunglasses

Americans buy 100,000,000 pairs of sunglasses each year, registering a $300,000,000-a-year market. The use of some sort of light filter is not unique to humans. Many fish have yellow pigment, often concentrated in the upper half of the cornea, that functions as a sort of eyeshade.[10] As for humans, we know that Turbenville of Salsbury, England, a famous 15th century ophthalmologist, prescribed silk veils for his postoperative patients who complained of hypersensitivity to light *(photophobia).*
Do sunglasses simply make vision more comfortable in very bright light, or do they actually improve vision? Our experiments suggest that in overbright conditions (beach, mountain tops, or on the water) we see better with sunglasses.[11] It has also been shown that spending all day at the beach under the summer sun without sunglasses will reduce visual sensitivity to 50% of normal at dusk. The dark adaptation mechanism suffers from prolonged exposure to bright light and may not completely return for a day or two.
The lens of the eye not only focuses objects on the retina, but also filters out visually annoying long ultraviolet light (wavelengths 310–390 nm). When the lens of the eye is removed surgically, as in cataract operations, spectacles not only must replace the optical power of the eye lens, but also must remove the blue end of the spectrum; this is accomplished with a sunglass filter. Polarizing sunglasses offer an added advantage over conventional sunglasses. They can actually improve visibility by eliminating glare from annoying reflecting surfaces.
Generally, the actual color of the spectacle lens does not affect vision, except in the case of the color-deficient patient. Here, the color should be pale or gray to avoid accentuating color deficiency.

References

1. Kupfer C: All about your eyes and how to save them. U.S. News and World Report 74 (24):66, 1973

2. Soresby A: Epidemiology of refraction. Int Ophthalmol Clin 11:1, 1971

3. Young F: Refractive errors, reading performances and school achievement among Eskimo children. Am J Optom 47:384, 1970

4. Baldwin W: A series study of refractive status in youth. Am J Optom 34:486, 1957

5. Young F: Pulman study: visual study of schoolchildren. Am J Optom 31:111, 1954

6. Donders FC: *On the Anomalies of Accommodation and Refraction of the Eye.* London, The New Sydenham Society, 1864

7. Miller D, Johnson R: Quantification of the pinhole effect. Surv Ophthalmol 21:347, 1977

8. Walsh FB, Hoyt WF: *Sensory Innervation of the Eye and Orbit,* 3d ed. Baltimore, Williams & Wilkins, 1969, p 423

9. Cameron ME: Headaches in relation to the eyes. Med J Aust 1:292, 1976

10. Moreland JD, Lythgoe JN: Yellow corneas in fishes. Vision Res 8:1377, 1968

11. Miller D: The effect of sunglasses on the visual mechanism. Surv Ophthalmol 19:38, 1974

Chapter 6

Contact Lenses

Contact lenses are small, corrective lenses worn immediately next to the cornea of the eye. Although eye specialists had been fitting special types of contact lenses to a limited number of patients for 100 years, the introduction of the "hard" corneal contact lens in 1948 was a major advance. The presently more popular "soft" lens, which was not developed in this country until 1966, was a similar milestone. Another type of contact lens, now largely supplanted by the corneal lenses, is the scleral lens, which was developed before 1900 but which still has several useful applications.

Hard Corneal Lenses

Typically 7–10 mm in diameter, hard contact lenses are made of a hard plastic—polymethyl methacrylate—that is very similar to Plexiglass (Fig. 6-1). Many of the problems originally associated with the fitting of patients with hard lenses have been eliminated over the past 30 years. Nevertheless, only 50% of those fitted with hard corneal lenses continue to wear them.[1] The major reason reported for discarding contact lenses is discomfort, as many have difficulty adapting to the presence of a hard foreign body on the eye that interferes with the flow of atmospheric oxygen to the cornea.

Soft Corneal Lenses

A soft hydrophilic contact lens made of hydroxyethyl methacrylate originated in Czechoslovakia in 1960.[2] An improved version of the soft

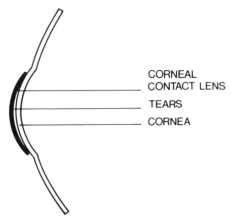

CORNEAL
CONTACT LENS
TEARS
CORNEA

Figure 6-1. Diagram showing how the tears are trapped by a corneal contact lens. (Artist: Laurel Cook.)

lens was introduced in the United States in 1966. Because of the plastic's ability to absorb moisture from the eye and to conform to the contour of the eye, these lenses cause little or no discomfort to the eye. Since the lens is soft and tends to assume the shape of the cornea, however, it does not correct significantly for high degrees of corneal distortion or for greater than 2 D of astigmatism.

There are a number of unique therapeutic applications of the soft lens—it can be used as a splint for slow-healing corneal epithelial defects and as a screen to protect against irritating, inturned lashes and to relieve the painful rubbing of the lids on a roughened or sensitive cornea. Soft lenses can also be used in conjunction with artificial tears to treat dry eyes. Since the lens can absorb certain medications, and then slowly deliver them to the eye over a 24-hour period, research is now in progress to see if eye medications can be more effectively applied by using soft lenses than by using conventional eyedrops.

An accurate applanation tonometry measurement of intraocular pressure can be performed on a cornea wearing a thin, relatively low-power soft lens. This consideration may be important for those who must wear continuous-wear, therapeutic soft lenses.

Benefits and Precautions

Since soft lenses are initially more comfortable to wear, and because the adaptation period is so much shorter than that for hard lenses, patients are sometimes tempted to wear their contact lenses too long. The soft plastic does not, however, perfectly transmit all the nutritive fluids and oxygen that the cornea needs, and patients should be advised to wear soft contacts as carefully as they would wear hard lenses. (In the long run, there is no evidence that soft lenses are more comfortable than properly fitted hard lenses after adaptation.)

Because of the chemical composition of *hydroxyethyl methacrylate*, bacteria tend to adhere more firmly to the surface of the soft lenses. As a result, patients must be cautioned to use appropriate solutions and to sterilize their lenses *nightly*. It is an absolute necessity to store soft lenses in solution, for otherwise they lose their water content and become irreversibly brittle. Soft lenses must also be handled carefully; they tear quite easily.

A bothersome condition seen with greater frequency as soft lenses are worn by more patients is *giant papillary conjunctivitis*. If ocular secretions are not thoroughly removed from the soft lens nightly, the secretions tend to build up and change in character so as to challenge allergically the inner surface of the upper lid. The palpebral conjunctiva of the upper lid becomes irritated and inflamed and develops large papules filled with lymphocytes and plasma cells. In order to continue to wear soft lenses, the patient must get fresh lenses or have the old lenses thoroughly cleaned.

Soft lenses will also absorb any aqueous solution. This can complicate matters if eyedrops must be prescribed for a soft-lens wearer. The lenses absorb the eyedrops and hold the drugs against the corneal tissue. Despite these complications, the benefits of soft lenses are clear.

To date, two groups in particular have benefited most from the introduction of soft contact lenses. Because they are more comfortable initially, people with very sensitive eyes are often able to adapt to soft lenses after failing to tolerate hard lenses. Soft lenses have been a great boon to athletes with refractive errors. Because the soft lenses are larger and hug the cornea more tightly, they are much less likely to be jarred loose than hard lenses, and, in addition, the soft lenses are far more comfortable to wear than scleral lenses, the athletes' other alternative. To these two groups, as well as to others, the extra cost of soft lenses is well worthwhile.

Scleral Lenses

These are large, hard lenses made of *polymethyl methacrylate* (Fig. 6-2) that cover the cornea and the entire sclera (white of the eye). Scleral lenses may be used when the cornea is so severely distorted that small corneal lenses will not stay in place. There are other applications as well.

In some eye diseases, the patient does not secrete enough tears to keep ahead of evaporation, or the lids do not moisten the corneas properly. In such cases, the corneas dry and lose their transparency. The use of scleral lenses, combined with artificial tears in drop form, keeps fluid in contact with the corneas.

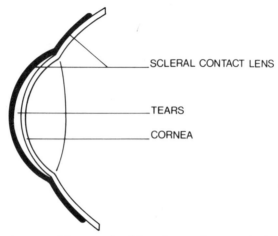

SCLERAL CONTACT LENS

TEARS

CORNEA

Figure 6-2. Diagram of how a scleral lens fits on the eye. (Artist: Laurel Cook.)

Scleral lenses are also used as splints for patients whose eyes have sustained chemical or thermal burns. The large scleral lens functions as a barrier in preventing adhesion between lid and eye during healing.

In all of the above situations, the scleral lenses are usually constructed from a plaster mold of the eye to be treated. Thus, the task of making and fitting scleral lenses is time-consuming. In general, most of the conditions that traditionally had been treated with scleral lenses are now treated with large soft contact lenses.

Bifocal Lenses

Many people beyond their midforties need reading glasses, or wear bifocals to correct presbyopia. Contact lenses can also be made in bifocal form. Fitting them is difficult, and the chances of success are not as great as with conventional contact lenses. One bifocal design recognizes that most people lower their eyes to read; the lens is made so that it rests on the margin of the lower lid. When its wearer looks down, the lens shifts its position on the cornea in relation to the pupil so that a person is looking through the lower portion of the contact, which is ground with a near-vision prescription. Another type of bifocal makes use of a multifocal lens; at any one time, objects at various distances are in focus, and the brain pays attention to the one of immediate importance.

Optics of Contact Lenses

In myopia, as explained in Chapter 5, the optical elements of the eye are too powerful for the size of the eye, and the image is focused in front of the retina. When proper contact lenses are fitted, the refracting power of the cornea is weakened sufficiently by substituting the front surface of the contact lens for the front surface of the cornea, and the image is then focused on the retina. Only trained ophthalmologists and optometrists can make the calculations required to achieve this precise substitution.

In hyperopia, the situation is the opposite of that in myopia. The optics of the eye are too weak, and the image is focused in back of the retina. The proper contact lens increases the converging power of the hyperopic cornea and brings the focus onto the retina.

In astigmatism, the cornea is imperfectly spherical, and all distance vision is distorted. When contacts are fitted, the rear surface of the lens traps the tear fluid between itself and the cornea, filling the misshapen areas. The perfectly spherical surface of the contact lens forms undistorted images on the retina. If an individual is also nearsighted or farsighted, the proper prescription is ground on the front surface of the contact lens.

How Contact Lenses Stay in Place

With corneal contact lenses, the presence of a tear film over the surface of the cornea helps to hold the lenses on the eye.[3] The surface tension of the tears function as a bridge that links the lens to the eye's surface.

Fitting the Contact Lens

The contact-lens fitter must meet four criteria to achieve a successful fit. The lens design must allow the oxygen-saturated tears to circulate effectively under the lens; the pressure of the lens on the eye must be evenly distributed; the lens must center properly over the pupil; and the proper refractive correction for the patient must be calculated. Fitting usually requires three to six visits, but some doctors spend one entire day with a patient and achieve a satisfactory fit without further visits.

Helping the Patient Adjust

Adaptation to the hard corneal lenses usually involves a few weeks of irritation and inconvenience. Since the lens is a foreign substance, the wearer initially senses the presence of a foreign body. A tolerance soon develops, however, so that the patient is hardly aware of the lenses' presence. Adaptation to the soft lens is often immediate.

Most doctors recommend a gradual breaking-in period. The patient usually starts wearing the lenses one or two hours a day, gradually increasing wearing time. The wearer must mesh this early adaptation schedule with his or her working schedule. Some doctors feel it is not necessary to reach all-day wear slowly, and have their patients begin immediately to wear their lenses all day.

There is no way of predicting, with 100% accuracy, whether a person will be able to wear contact lenses successfully. The only sure way to find out is to attempt a fitting. About 70% of those patients who obtain a proper fitting are able to wear hard contact lenses.[1] The success rate increases to over 90% with soft contact lenses.[4]

A survey of wearers in the United States showed that the 50% of people fitted with hard contact lenses who continued to wear their lenses fall into three major categories: people who see much better with contact lenses than with glasses; highly motivated people who feel that the advantage of improved appearance overrides the discomforts and annoyances that often accompany contact-lens wear; and very careful people who have perfectly fitted lenses and do not overwear their lenses. The study listed the four most common reasons patients offered for giving up their contacts: discomfort, too much bother, loss of lens, and corneal ulcers from wearing the lenses.[1]

Eye Damage from Contact Lenses

In March 1966 a report based on the records of nearly 50,000 hard contact-lens wearers appeared in the Journal of the American Medical Association. Of these patients, 14 eyes had been lost or blinded as a direct result of wearing contact lenses; 157 other eyes were permanently damaged, and 7,607 eyes suffered reversible, but serious, damage.[5]

Causes

The same study showed that most permanent damage occurred when contact-lens wearers wore their lenses continually for days, or even weeks, in the presence of corneal infection or in spite of symptoms of overwear or poor fit. The major risk in contact-lens wear is that the lens will scratch the cornea, and that the scratch will then become infected. The cornea can be scratched if the lens is worn for too long, if it is inserted carelessly, or if a small foreign body gets blown under the lens and is rubbed into the corneal surface.

Symptoms and Treatment of
Contact-Lens-Related Corneal Abrasion

A corneal abrasion caused by a contact lens is not something that most patients will be able to ignore. The eye reddens suddenly, and burns or hurts, even after the lenses are removed. Vision in the affected eye may be hazy, and the eye may be photophobic, both symptoms persist after the lens is removed. In some cases, pain and other symptoms do not develop while the lenses are in place, but occur several hours after the lenses have been removed. Treatment consists of removing the lenses and proscribing their use until the ulcer has healed. The physician should attempt to determine the cause of the abrasion (careless insertion, wind-blown foreign matter, prolonged wear). First aid should be administered for corneal abrasion as described in Chapter 13.

Prevention

Rules for the Lens Wearer. Thè first step in the prevention of eye damage is to prevent corneal scratches (also called corneal abrasions or ulcers).

1. The lenses must be smooth. If they have a rough surface or are chipped, they must not be worn and should be replaced immediately.

2. The lenses should be inserted in a clean, quiet place, and should not be rushed.

3. Dirty or dusty conditions should be avoided. In wind, the patient should wear protective glasses such as sunglasses.

4. Identification of right and left lenses is crucial if the lenses are different; blurred vision immediately subsequent to insertion may be due to switched lenses.

If vision remains unclear for more than half an hour after the patient removes his or her contact lenses and puts on glasses with a current prescription, the patient is suffering from a condition known as *spectacles blur.* The contact lenses have altered the surface of the cornea; this is an indication that refitting is necessary.

Care of Hard Contact Lenses. Proper care of contact lenses can contribute to prevention of corneal abrasions and infections. Wetting solutions are used to insure that tears will circulate evenly over and around the lenses as soon as they are inserted, thus helping to maintain a steady supply of moisture and oxygen to the corneas. Many wetting solutions also contain a preservative to help reduce the chances of bacteria being introduced into the eye along with the lens.

Cleaning solutions should be used periodically because the mucous component of tears tends to build up on contact lenses with time. If the mucous is allowed to accumulate and harden over a period of weeks, it will create a cloudy layer over the lens surface that interferes with vision.

Most ophthalmologists prefer that their patients soak their lenses overnight in storage solutions. These preparations have some of the properties of both wetting and cleaning solutions; they prevent the build-up of residue and make insertion more comfortable.

Lens loss is a fairly common occurrence during the first three years of wear, especially with hard corneal lenses. It has been estimated that upwards of 70% of contact-lens wearers will lose one or more lenses during this period. It is considered advisable to obtain replacements from the physician or optometrist who originally fitted the lenses.

Indications and Contraindications for Contact Lenses

Roughly 10 million Americans use contact lenses. This figure is increasing by more than 10% each year. Of those patients wearing contact lenses, about 80% are female and 20% are male. Most contact-lens wearers are in their midteens to midtwenties. However, children younger than 4 and adults over 80 are successfully wearing contact lenses. It has been estimated that almost 90% of those who wear contact lenses do so because they feel that spectacles detract from their appearance.

Athletics

The athlete who wears eyeglasses is faced with the problems of mist, rain, dust, ice, snow, or mud on his lenses, poor peripheral vision, and the danger of being seriously hurt if hit on the face while wearing glasses. Consequently, professional athletes in almost all the major sports wear contact lenses. Swimming is an exception (unless the swimmer wears tightly fitting goggles) since water neutralizes the adhering pressures that keep the lenses in place. Special contact lenses can be made for swimmers.

Cataract Removal

After cataract surgery, the eye requires a large amount of converging power to focus properly. People who have undergone cataract surgery usually must wear thick magnifying glasses. Aside from being heavy to wear and unsightly, these glasses introduce a number of optical defects: side vision is distorted and a portion of the side vision is actually blocked out; and the glasses magnify everything by about 25% to 30%, so that things appear abnormally large and unreal.

The patient who has had a cataract removed from one eye and who has normal vision in his other eye is faced with still another problem if he attempts to wear spectacles in front of the operated eye. Everything appears magnified to the operated eye, and normal to the good eye. The brain becomes confused by the different messages sent from each eye, and the patient frequently complains of dizziness and loss of equilibrium. A contact-lens correction after cataract surgery allows for more natural vision. Side vision is normal and very little magnification is introduced. According to most medical experts, a contact lens can be fitted safely 12 to 16 weeks after cataract surgery.

Distorted Corneas

The cornea is so important in focusing that it is easy to appreciate how a misshapen or washboard-surfaced cornea makes focusing impossible, even with spectacles. Irregular corneas are often caused by scarring that follows severe corneal infections or injuries. *Keratoconus* is a type of corneal distortion in which the cornea assumes the shape of a cone. In some advanced cases, the cornea comes almost to a point (Fig. 6-3). Its cause is unknown, but it is believed that it may be a hereditary condition.

The solution to the problem of corrected distorted corneas was first suggested by Leonardo da Vinci in 1508.[6] In his *Codex of the Eye,* he noted that he could neutralize the focusing properties of the cornea with a water-containing lens held against the eye. The present-day contact lens works in a similar manner. Our tears, which are essentially like water, have optical properties very similar to those of the cornea, and a contact lens helps hold this fluid in place to fill in or surround the corneal irregularities (Fig. 6-1).

Changing Eye Color

Our eyes are considered blue or brown or hazel because that is the color of the iris. In the 1940s, Walter Hampden, a blue-eyed actor, convincingly played the part of an American Indian only with the aid of a contact lens in which the portion over his iris was tinted brown.[7] Such lenses are now available for the general public, but fittings are difficult, because the colored portion of the lens must center perfectly over the patient's own iris.

Special Problem Groups

Most healthy people who are not overly sensitive about putting something in their eye will be able to wear contact lenses. A number of situations, however, make wearing conventional contact lenses more difficult.

Dry Eyes. Since the contact lens essentially floats on a layer of tears, absence of tears means that the lens must sit on the corneal surface directly. Thus, with each blink or eye movement, the cornea is scraped by the lens, causing pain and damage. Many of these patients can wear soft lenses, however, if they use artificial tears frequently to keep the lens and cornea moist.

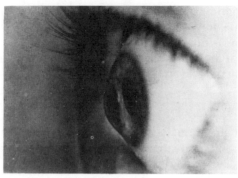

Figure 6-3. Profile of a cornea with keratoconus.

Severe Arthritis. Patients with severe arthritis of the fingers often cannot manipulate such small objects as contact lenses. Even if they are able to hold the lenses, arthritics may have great difficulty in placing them in their eyes.

Hay Fever and Other Allergies. These patients usually tolerate lenses well until allergy season rolls around. Then their eyes itch and run, and the presence of such foreign bodies as contact lenses is often intolerable.

Pregnancy. A woman fitted with contact lenses before she becomes pregnant often has trouble wearing them during pregnancy. The complete reason for this is unknown, but it appears that in some cases the hormones that circulate at high levels through the pregnant woman's body tend to produce lid edema, to alter tear characteristics, and even to alter the oxygen demand of the cornea. If these changes occur, the lenses do not fit properly. When the pregnancy is over, the woman usually can resume wearing her lenses.

Oral Contraception. The hormones of most contraceptive medications produce many of the changes seen in pregnancy, and thus cause contact lenses to fit poorly. A woman who plans to take the "pill" for some time should be fitted for contact lenses after her doctor feels she has been stabilized on the pill.

Epilepsy. Epileptic patients tolerate contact lenses, but if they should suffer a prolonged fit of unconsciousness, the contact lens may stay on the cornea for too long a time and cause damage. These patients should carry some form of identification that informs physicians or other emergency personnel that they have epilepsy and are wearing contact lenses.

Bifocals. Some patients need two prescriptions, one for distance vision and one for near vision. To accomplish this with contact lenses, the ophthalmologist has three choices: prescribe contact lenses for distance vision and glasses for reading; prescribe contact lenses with a reading prescription for one eye and a distance prescription for the other eye; or prescribe multifocal contact lenses (i.e., bifocal or *aspheric* lenses).

Work under Dirty, Dusty Conditions. People who work in mines, in textile or paper mills, or with drills or sandblasters run the risk of getting small particles under the contact lens. The lens has a tendency to rub these particles into the cornea, producing dangerous scratches that can become infected.

New Developments

Since softness is obviously important for comfort, other soft plastics are now being investigated. One such plastic is *silicone.* This plastic contains no water and therefore cannot dry out. It is readily tolerated by the body, and has been used in plastic and reconstructive surgery and to manufacture artificial heart valves. Since silicone is highly oxygen-permeable, a silicone contact lens allows direct gas-exchange through it to the cornea.

Now that polymer chemists know that softness, clarity, and oxygen permeability are important properties of a contact lens, we can expect a number of new types of contact lenses to appear on the market. It may not be too far-fetched to envision the day when contact lenses will be worn comfortably and never have to be removed.

Since hard lenses offer superior optics, research in the development of oxygen-permeable hard lenses continues. Among the promising new hard plastics are *cellulose acetate butyrate (CAB)* and combinations of *silicone* and *polymethyl methacrylate.*

Questions Patients Commonly Ask about Contact Lenses

Can contact lenses stop the progression of myopia?

A number of ophthalmologists have reported instances in which the progression of nearsightedness seemed to stop once contact lenses were applied. It is difficult to evaluate such claims because myopia often stops progressing on its own. Until controlled studies prove that myopic progression can be halted by contact lenses, and no other factor, this claim is open to suspicion.

Can contact lenses stop the progression of keratoconus?

Here again, we are dealing with a condition that sometimes halts by itself. It is not surprising that contact (particularly scleral) lenses have been given credit for stopping a condition that may have stopped on its own. Studies in which precise molds of the eye were periodically made demonstrated that keratoconus still progressed, even though scleral contact lenses were being worn.

Can contact lenses become lost in the eye?

A contact lens may slip under the upper or lower lid, but it can always be recovered easily by its wearer. A contact lens can *never* get behind the eye or into the eye itself.

Are there contact lenses that never touch the eye?

Statements to this effect have appeared in certain contact lens advertisements, and, of course, in a strict sense, they are true. The contact lens rests on the eye, but if the lens is fitted properly, it will actually be floating on a microscopically thin layer of tears.

Can you go to sleep with your contacts in?

Research still needs to be done in this area, and it may one day be possible to sleep while wearing soft lenses. It is definitely not safe to sleep while wearing conventional hard or soft lenses, because very little oxygen can reach the cornea when the lid is closed and the lens inserted.

I've heard that you can't wear cosmetics if you wear contacts.

Untrue, but certain brands and types of cosmetics and sprays are more likely to get into the eyes while wearing contact lenses.

Can certain contact lenses bring the eyes back to normality?

It has been known for a long time that a poorly fitting contact lens causes the cornea to swell and change shape. Often this pathologic swelling causes the cornea to flatten slightly and to lose some converging power. Such a change may improve myopic vision, but there are serious drawbacks. First, cutting off the oxygen supply to induce corneal swelling can lead to serious corneal damage. Second, even if the desired corneal change is achieved, once the contact lens is removed, the healthy cornea will return to its original shape in a few weeks or months.

The Choice between Soft and Hard Lenses

This is a decision made by the eye doctor after a thorough history and eye examination. The following factors will determine the final decision.

Astigmatism. Patients with more than 1.5 to 2.0 D of astigmatism do not see well with soft contact lenses.

Cataract Surgery. Most of these patients require strong plus lens prescriptions. Such powers are more accurately made in hard lenses.

Keratoconus, Distorted Corneas. Since soft lenses tend to fit cornea deformities in a "hand-and-glove" manner, hard lenses will neutralize these optical defects more efficiently.

Discomfort Tolerance. Hard lenses are initially more uncomfortable than soft lenses, and so patients who cannot tolerate the initial discomfort of hard lenses should try soft lenses.

Self-Discipline. Soft lenses are fragile and require a nightly discipline of cleaning and disinfection. Certain personalities can tolerate such a regimen better than others.

Allergic History. Either lens may be uncomfortable during the patient's allergic season, but soft lenses tend to concentrate more airborne allergen than hard lenses.

Cost. Soft lenses tend to be more expensive on initial purchase, and replacement of soft lenses also tends to be more expensive than hard lenses.

Sports Use. Soft lenses tend to stay on the eye better than hard lenses during vigorous athletic activities.

Eye Dryness. Both types of lenses need to ride on a bed of tears. Soft lenses also need fluid to remain hydrated and to retain their original shape. Thus, soft lenses on a dry eye will need frequent applications of artificial tears to remain comfortable.

Corneal Abrasion History. A patient with a history of frequent corneal abrasions connected with the use of hard lenses should try soft lenses.

References

1. Sarver M, Harris MG: A standard for success in wearing contact lenses. Am J Optom 48:382, 1971

2. Wichterle O, Lin D: Hydrophilic gels for biological use. Nature 185:117, 1960

3. Miller D: An analysis of the physical forces applied to a corneal contact lens. Arch Ophthalmol 70:823, 1963

4. Soft-con Corrective Lens Study: Evaluation by slit-lamp and patient symptoms. Warner-Lambert, Nov 1974, pp 1–5

5. Dixon JM, Young CA, Baldone JA, et al: Committee on contact lens report. JAMA 195:901, 1966

6. Mandell RB: *Contact Lens Practice.* Springfield, Ill, Thomas, 1965, p 3

7. Baker J: *The Truth About Contact Lenses.* New York, Putnam, 1970, p 19

Chapter 7

Response of the Cornea to Disease

When jobs were assigned to the parts of the body, the human cornea was given a difficult task: to be the major refracting element of the eye (three times as powerful as the crystalline lens), to be perfectly clear (without blood vessels), and to maintain a flawless optical surface despite exposure to the environment. To accomplish its three-part task, the cornea is divided into three major zones. The epithelial cells maintain surface smoothness and clarity; the stroma insures structural integrity and optical curvature; and the endothelial layer is the primary regulator of the nutritional supply (Fig. 7-1). The strange and wonderful thing is that these three components have been designed to do their jobs and also to remain transparent. If one of these zones is the subject of a disease process, however, its transparency is compromised and an opacity develops. With the aid of a slit lamp, the corneal expert can look at a cornea, locate the zone of pathology, describe the pattern of opacity, and, more often than not, determine the cause of the problem.

In this chapter, I will describe some of the unique features of each of these zones and their characteristic disease patterns.

The Corneal Epithelium

Structure and Function

To remain transparent, the five layers of cells must be bound together to produce a sheet of uniform refractive index. In order to prevent fluid of refractive index different from that of the cell cytoplasm from seeping between cell borders, a system of tight junctions and *zonula occludens* keeps

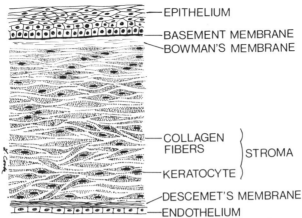

EPITHELIUM
BASEMENT MEMBRANE
BOWMAN'S MEMBRANE

COLLAGEN
FIBERS   } STROMA
KERATOCYTE

DESCEMET'S MEMBRANE
ENDOTHELIUM

Figure 7-1. Drawing of a histologic section of the cornea. (Artist: Laurel Cook.)

the cells no more than 100μ apart.[1] If the intraocular pressure should rise sharply, as it does in glaucoma, aqueous is forced through the stroma and lodges between the epithelial cells (Fig. 7-2). To the observer, the epithelial zone then looks like a sheet of ground glass because the optical mismatch of edema fluid and cells backscatters the examiner's light. The edematous epithelium acts as a diffraction grating, and so when looking at a small light the patient sees an interference pattern that looks like a halo.[2]

The tight cellular junctions also prevent the tears and their chemical constituents from penetrating the epithelium and disrupting its clarity. If toxic chemicals such as lye, cleaning solvents, or acids are splashed into the eye, however, many of the surface cells are either destroyed or damaged. Under slit-lamp examination, superficial punctate opacities mark the scattered sites of epithelial swelling and protein denaturation. The scattered-dot pattern assumes a glowing yellow-green color when a drop of fluorescein is instilled into the eye and illuminated by the blue light of the slit lamp. The water-soluble dye works by seeping through or around the damaged cells and staining the underlying stroma.[1,3]

Abrasions

Unlike skin epithelium, the corneal epithelium normally is not covered by translucent, leathery keratin, and therefore it is vulnerable to the scrapes and nicks of wind-blown particles, fingernails, paper edges, and the like. Fingernails and paper edges characteristically produce epithelial damage that appears in a dotted-gray, linear pattern when viewed through the slit lamp. When wind-blown particles strike the eye, they often become trapped in the succulent undersurface of the upper lid, carving vertical linear abrasions with each blink of the lid.

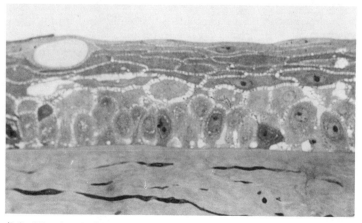

Figure 7-2. Histology of edematous epithelium: note the rings of edema fluid surrounding the epithelial cells. (Courtesy of T. Kuwabara and reprinted with permission from Miller D, Benedek G: *Intraocular Light Scattering.* Springfield, Ill., Thomas, 1973, p 54.)

Infection

Unlike the neighboring epithelial cells of the conjunctiva, which are prone to infection (conjunctivitis is a common condition caused by a multitude of bacteria and viruses), the healthy corneal epithelium is resistant to all but a few organisms (e.g., *Neisseria gonorrhoeae, Chlamidia trachomatis,* herpes simplex, herpes [varicella-] zoster, and adenovirus). The most common ocular viral infection in America is herpes simplex keratitis. Herpetic infection is believed to result from the activation of the dormant virus, which probably resides in the Gasserian ganglion and along the fifth nerve.[4] It is not known what activates the virus or compromises corneal resistance, but physical trauma, fever, or local instillation of epinephrine or steroids can activate the dormant virus in animals and man.[5] The herpes virus usually destroys the surface epithelium in a gray, dendritic pattern. With fluorescein instillation, the stroma below the diseased cells glow in the same dendritic shape (Fig. 7-3). In a case of superficial herpetic infection, treatment initially consists of frequent application of topical antiviral medication (idoxuridine or cytosine arabinoside). If the infection does not respond in a week, the entire corneal surface (containing epithelial cells and the resident viruses) is surgically debrided. The cornea usually resurfaces with healthy cells in a few days. If the virus infects the stroma, however, resolution of the inflammation may take many months and often eventuates in a corneal scar.

Cancer

The corneal epithelium is resistant not only to invasion by many microorganisms, but also to neoplastic changes. Neighboring conjunctival

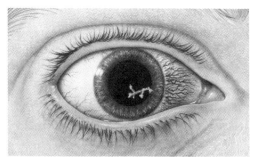

Figure 7-3. Drawing of a cornea with a dendritic ulcer.

epithelium, however, may convert to basal-cell or squamous-cell carcinoma.[6] The limbal epithelium also is vulnerable to carcinoma in situ (Bowen's disease). Nevertheless, cancer of the corneal epithelium has been reported only once, and then only over an area of scarred and vascularized stroma.[7]

Allergy

The cornea is also resistant to allergy. A patient who is allergic to ragweed pollen becomes a victim of the allergen after it passes between the loosely hinged epithelium of the conjunctiva and contacts a mast cell.[8] The tightly bound corneal epithelium allows few such molecules to pass. Even in the event of passage, there are no mast cells in the corneal stroma to interact with an allergen and induce inflammation.

There are instances, however, notably in herpes simplex infection, in which it is thought that the virus transforms the corneal stroma into antigenic complexes, which are then attacked by immunologic cells. Thus, one school of thought feels that treatment should consist of corticosteroids, to counteract the allergic response, and the appropriate antiviral medication, to eradicate any viable virus.

Ultraviolet Burns

Whereas the most efficient ultraviolet wavelength for the production of dermal erythema is 300 nm, the peak wavelength that incites ultraviolet keratitis is 288 nm.[9,10] This portion of the ultraviolet spectrum produces pyrimidine dimers in the nucleic acid portion of the DNA of the corneal epithelium.[11] Thus, if an eye is exposed to the ultraviolet radiation of a welding arc or a sun lamp, no symptoms are noted immediately. But within 12 hours the epithelial cells slowly swell, yielding a picture of many tiny granular opacities splattered over the corneal surface.[12] The process continues until the swollen cells burst and slough, producing zones of punctate pathology that take the fluorescein stain. Typically, the patient exposed to ultraviolet radiation in the afternoon goes to bed asymptomatic, and is awakened in the middle of the night with severe eye pain.

The patient turns on the light and discovers intense photophobia. The pain and photophobia are usually incapacitating, but slowly subside over the next 24 hours. No treatment other than mild analgesics is required, and the patient is left with no corneal sequelae.

Dryness

The corneal surface must be perpetually wetted to keep it smooth and clean and to prevent dryness, which can lead to keratinization and opacification. The normal cornea maintains a tear film 7μ thick.[13] The film is continually renewed by secretions from the lacrimal gland, *conjunctival goblet cells,* and *meibomian glands,* while old tears are flushed down the lacrimal puncta by the muscular action of the lids. If one of the fluid components (tear mucus, or lipids) is not supplied, or if the blink mechanism controlled by the seventh nerve fails to function, the wetting system cannot operate properly (Table 7-1). In all of the examples of improper corneal wetting described below, the drying occurs primarily on the lower cornea, the area not covered by the upper lid. Thus, clumps of gray, crenated cells dot the inferior third of the corneal surface in the pattern characteristic of exposure keratopathy.

In Sjögren's syndrome, lymphocytes attack the glands of the nasal, buccal, and vaginal mucosa, the synovia of the joints, and the lacrimal glands.[14] The lacrimal gland slowly atrophies, and the corneal surface dries from lack of tears. This drying produces punctate areas of epithelial death. With the epithelial barrier damaged or absent, bacterial ulceration of the stroma can occur. Prophylactic treatment consists of the use of artificial tears to keep the cornea moist.

Even though the corneal epithelium is normally hydrophobic (a drop of water will not spread across a cornea that has been wiped dry[15]), tears spread because of the wetting-agent action of the mucus. Mucus, secreted by the conjunctival goblet cells and held in place by villi from the corneal epithelium, is rubbed into the cornea during each blink. In erythema multiforme, the cornea dries because the conjunctival goblet cells are

Table 7-1. Conditions That Result in Dry Eyes

Condition	Causes
Decreased meibomian secretion	Scarring from chemical burns, erythema multiforme, ocular pemphigoid, old trachoma
Decreased aqueous phase	Congenital alacrima, neurogenic hyposecretion, Sjögren's syndrome
Decreased mucus	Avitaminosis; scarring from ocular pemphigoid, erythema multiforme, chemical burns, old trachoma

destroyed and there is a deficiency of conjunctival mucus.[16] In severe chemical burns of the eye and lids, the meibomian glands may fail to secrete sufficient lipids, and evaporation and loss of tears proceeds at an abnormally rapid rate, leading to a state of corneal drying.

Corneal dryness may also be caused by damage to the seventh nerve, as occurs in *Bell's palsy*. In this condition, the tears and mucus are produced, but the lids cannot function to spread tears over the cornea. The lower uncovered cornea dries, producing an inferior punctate pattern that often coalesces into an ulcer. Treatment consists of suturing the lids together laterally *(tarsorrhaphy)* so as to keep most of the cornea covered while allowing the patient to see through a crack. If the partial tarsorrhaphy does not keep the cornea completely moist, a soft contact lens fitted under the partially closed lid will maintain corneal integrity.

Although of little importance in the United States, *nutritional xerophthalmia*, which is caused by Vitamin A and protein deficiency, is a major cause of blindness worldwide. The lack of these nutrients in the diet reduces conjunctival mucus production, which leads to corneal drying, corneal keratinization, and thus corneal opacification.

The Stroma

Structure and Function

The refractive power of the cornea resides in the stroma, a fibrous structure with very few cells. The curvature of the developing stroma is determined in utero by three factors: the intraocular pressure, which causes the developing cornea to bulge outward; the resistance of the *limbal ring*, which does not yield to intraocular pressure;[17] and the rate at which the stroma is laid down and polymerized. The fibers of the stroma are tough and held together tightly in a very regular pattern by a mucopolysaccharide glue (Fig. 7-4). Because the glue consists mostly of water, which has a refractive index of 1.33, the distance between the fibers (index of refraction 1.47) is critical to corneal transparency. If this distance becomes greater than half a wavelength of light (as occurs in corneal edema), the cornea thickens, light-scattering increases, transparency is lost, and the cornea takes on a gray quality that progresses to white as the edema increases.[2,18]

Infection

In the event that the epithelial barrier is traumatized, accidental introduction of any one of many pathogenic bacteria into the eye can produce a localized ulcer. A staphylococcal ulcer, for example, produces a yellow-white opacity in the stroma and, upon histologic examination, shows

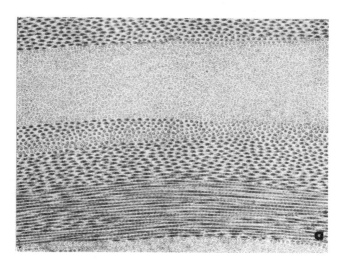

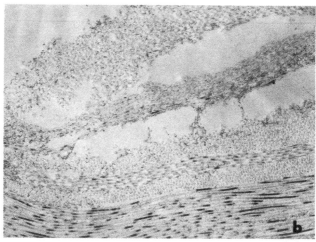

Figure 7-4. Electron micrograph of **a** normal versus **b** edematous stroma. (Note lakes of fluid in the edematous stroma in the lower photograph.) (Courtesy of T. Kuwabara and reprinted with permission from Miller D, Benedek G: *Intraocular Light Scattering.* Springfield, Ill., Thomas, 1973, p 20.)

heavy infiltration of inflammatory cells and fraying and dissolution of collagen fibers. The presence of both inflammatory cells and destroyed tissue causes large fluctuation in the refractive index of the stroma, resulting in intense reflection and backscatter of incident light that makes the ulcer opaque. Treatment of bacterial or fungal corneal ulcers involves the following steps: (1) scraping of the ulcer bed, (2) staining and culturing the specimen, (3) topically applying a broad-spectrum antibiotic (gentamicin) initially, and (4) instituting specific antibiotic treatment once the organism and its sensitivity are determined.

Keratoconus

In *keratoconus,* the epithelium is thought to secrete an enzyme that digests the anterior stroma; the cornea thins and the thinned area bulges, thereby distorting the corneal surface.[19] The disease usually begins when the patient is between the ages of 15 and 25 years,[19] and it generally stabilizes within 10 years.

The incidence of keratoconus in the general population is about 1.3 per 1,000.[19] Its incidence in atopic dermatitis patients is relatively high, and most patients with keratoconus have an elevated level of the immunoglobulin IgE.[20] In patients with mongolism, the incidence of keratoconus is approximately six percent.[21] Keratoconus can usually be corrected with a contact lens.

As the disease progresses, however, scar tissue accumulates in the areas of thinning.[22] These stromal scars contain randomly arranged collagen fibers whose diameters are five times the normal thickness.[23] Both the coarseness of the fibers and their random distribution result in increased light-scattering, and small vertical linear opacities develop in the central corneal stroma. If the scarring and surface irregularity progress to a point at which contact lenses produce little improvement in visual acuity, corneal transplantation becomes necessary.

Systemic Disease

In a number of systemic diseases, the corneal stroma becomes a repository for crystals and other organic accumulations. The crystals and other deposits disrupt the precise optic order of the stroma and produce opacity. Strangely enough, these different opacities occur in discrete corneal locations, and each has a characteristic pattern.

Calcium Bands. In conditions in which the plasma-calcium concentration is increased, such as in *primary hyperparathyroidism* or *sarcoidosis,*[24] calcium often precipitates in a thin white sheet just below the basal epithelial layer. The sheet usually starts at the *limbus,* in the 3 and 9 o'clock positions, and slowly advances in a bandlike fashion across the exposed central cornea.

Because the cornea does not have its own blood supply, its temperature is determined by that of the environment, the aqueous humor, and the periodic warmth contributed by the blinking lid. Since the upper and lower portions of the cornea are more apt to be covered by the lids, these areas are a few degrees warmer than the exposed central portion.[25] It seems reasonable, therefore, that the increased calcium leaving the perilimbal vessels precipitates in the cooler, exposed part of the cornea, producing the band. If the band extends across the corneal center, it can be dissolved by applying the chelating agent EDTA to the scraped corneal surface.

Gout. Band keratopathy is occasionally seen in patients with gout. In these cases, the urate crystals are deposited within the nuclei of epithelial cells, and so the band is more superficial than in calcific band keratopathy.[26] Again, if the crystals cover the central cornea, decreasing vision, they must be scraped away surgically.

Wilson's Disease (Hepatolenticular Degeneration). In patients with *Wilson's disease,* lack of the copper-binding protein *ceruloplasmin* leads to deposition of copper in the brain, liver, and cornea, in which it may form a *Kayser-Fleischer ring.* The ring, usually brown, starts at the superior limbus and progresses to encircle the entire limbus. The copper is apparently taken up from the aqueous component by the endothelial cells and deposited in *Descemet's membrane,* the basement membrane continually laid down by the endothelial cells, and located just posterior to the stromal limit.[27] The ring, which does not impair vision, is detected in 50% of those patients with Wilson's disease. It usually regresses after systemic treatment with penicillamine.

Arcus Senilis. In this condition, phospholipids accumulate throughout the entire thickness of stroma to form a ringlike opacity in the peripheral cornea. Known as *arcus senilis,* this condition leaves a clear zone of about 1 mm between the fat deposits and the limbus. Arcus senilis is an inherited autosomal dominant trait and is sometimes associated with familial hypercholesterolemia and atherosclerosis.[28] The phospholipids leak out of the perilimbal capillaries and seep between the collagen fibers, spreading them apart and disrupting their transparent configuration to produce the characteristic white-ring opacity.

Cystinosis. In *cystinosis,* yellow-brown crystals of cystine may be deposited between the collagen fibers in the anterior stroma.[29,30] A general corneal haze is produced because the refractive index of the crystals differs from that of the surrounding cornea. Nevertheless, vision is usually not impaired. These crystals are sometimes removed by a superficial keratectomy. Occasionally, a similar configuration of corneal crystals are present throughout the entire stromal thickness.

See Table 7-2 for a list of systemic diseases that affect the stroma.

The Endothelium

Structure and Function

As mentioned earlier, excessive fluid impairs corneal transparency. Yet the cells of the stroma and epithelium need the nutrition and fluid provided by the aqueous humor. It is the job of the endothelial layer

Table 7-2. Systemic Diseases That Produce Stromal Abnormalities

Disease	Finding	Localization	Local Treatment
Hyperparathyroidism, sarcoidosis	Calcium-band keratopathy	Below basal epithelium, 3–9 o'clock	EDTA
Gout	Urate-band keratopathy	Epithelial cell nuclei	Surgical scraping
Wilson's disease	Kayser-Fleischer ring keratopathy	Perilimbal brown ring in Descemet's membrane	Penicillamine
Arcus senilis	Ring opacity (white) in simple cornea	Throughout stroma	No treatment needed
Cystinosis	Cystine crystals—corneal haze (yellow brown)	Anterior stroma	Superficial keratectomy

(which consists of just one layer of cells) to allow the aqueous component into the cornea and to pump out excess fluid so that transparency is maintained.[31] The pump seems to be of the Na-K-ATPase variety, and is located in the cell membranes of the endothelium.[32]

The endothelial cells are hexagonal in shape, and seem fitted together much as tiles on a floor. The hexagonal configuration, just as in a beehive, minimizes mechanical stress between units.

Trauma

Physical trauma of the type that may occur during a cataract extraction or an infection from herpes virus can temporarily interfere with the pump. The pump is also progressively and permanently weakened in an inherited disorder known as *Fuchs' corneal endothelial dystrophy.*[33,34] In all of the above circumstances, if sufficient fluid is not pumped out, the cornea thickens and its transparency is compromised, giving the cornea a generally hazy-gray appearance. If the edema does not reverse itself, a corneal transplant is the proper treatment.

Iritis

In patients with *iritis,* white cells are deposited into the anterior chamber. Gray-white clumps of these cells, visible with the slit lamp, often stick to the endothelial surface of the cornea. Cells within these keratitic precipitates send out pseudopods that are inserted between endothelial cells.[35] The pseudopods create spaces through which the aqueous humor can flow into the stroma and cause local corneal edema. When the iritis responds to therapy (usually topical steroids), the precipitates melt away and the edema resolves.

Corneal Transplantation

If the cornea's response to disease results in loss of its transparency by scarring or edema, corneal transplantation becomes the proper treatment. In 1907, the first successful transplantation of a human cornea was performed by a Czechoslovakian surgeon, Edward Zirm.[36] The recipient was a 45-year-old laborer who had had hot lime splashed in both eyes 15 months before surgery. The donor was an 11-year-old boy whose right eye was removed because of an injury. Since the boy's cornea had not been injured, Zirm removed a central disc and attached it over a corresponding hole made in the recipient's eye.

Since then, corneal transplantation has become a common procedure with an overall success rate of about 75% (see Figs. 7-5, 7-6, 7-7). Nevertheless, the chances of success vary with the underlying pathologic

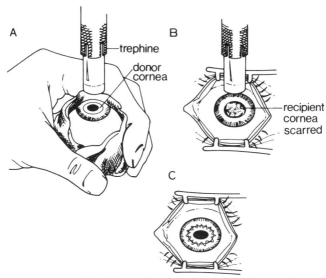

Figure 7-5. Diagram showing the major steps in a corneal transplant operation. (Artists: David Lobel, Laurel Cook.)

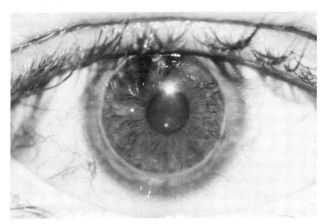

Figure 7-6. Photograph of a cornea with a clear transplant.

conditions: for keratoconus, it may be as high as 90%; for an alkali-burned cornea, it may be as low as 25%.[37] Since the recipient's cells eventually replace the transplanted epithelial and stromal cells, the key to success lies in the state of health of the transplanted endothelial cells, which are not replaced by host cells; graft failure can result from unsuitable storage of donor tissue, dystrophy of the donor's endothelium, surgical trauma, or immunologic rejection of the endothelium.[38] During immunologic attack, lymphocytes invade the endothelium, capillaries and lymphatics invade the stroma, and antibodies precipitate antigens in the

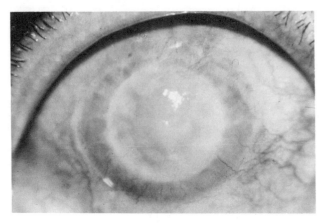

Figure 7-7. Photograph of a rejected corneal transplant.

stroma,[39] all of which cloud the transplanted cornea. Impending rejection is usually treated with heavy doses of topical steroids. If this treatment fails (Fig. 7-6, bottom), a new cornea may be transplanted again. In one patient, more than 20 grafts were performed before success was achieved.

Because of the cornea's avascularity, good results in corneal transplantation do not require such precautions as tissue-typing, which are needed for other types of grafts. If a transplanted cornea is not compatible with the refractive error of the recipient's eyes, glasses or contact lenses provide clear vision.

Eye Banks

Most large cities have eye banks. If you know of someone interested in donating their eyes upon death for use in corneal transplantation, ask the local eye bank for donation blanks.

Facts for Eye Donors

Eye surgeons estimate that several thousands of needlessly blind persons could be helped to regain their sight through the corneal transplant operation. Thus, public awareness of the following facts about donating eyes should be promoted:

1. There are no age limits for donors.

2. Wearing of glasses, most previous eye surgery, or eye diseases do not prevent one from becoming a donor.

3. Eyes must be removed as soon as possible after the donor's death and may be kept for as long as 48 hours.

4. There is no disfigurement after the removal of donated eyes.

5. Since donated eyes must be removed under sterile conditions as soon as possible, it is presently practical to obtain eyes only from persons who die in a hospital.

6. There are no religious objections on the part of the Protestant, Catholic, or Jewish faiths to the donation of eyes.*

7. Eye banks reserve the right to determine the purposes for which the eye tissue will be used, but no eye is ever wasted. Eyes that for technical reasons are unsuitable for transplant are invaluable for research. Someday the knowledge gained from research may contribute to the cure and prevention of many causes of blindness.

Summary of Corneal Diseases

The diagnoses of corneal diseases are the result of analysis of three factors:

1. The presence of an opacity suggests a disease process.

2. Use of the slit lamp establishes the corneal zone in which the opacity is located, and determines whether it is an active process or an old inactive scar.

3. Third, the geographic distribution of the opacity, as well as the affected corneal zone, team up to suggest the cause of the disease.

References

1. Liegel O: Elektronenmikoskopische Untersuchungen über die Fluoresceinbarriere am intakten Hornhautepithel. Dtsch Ophthalmol Ges Berl 68:220, 1968

2. Miller D, Benedek G: *Intraocular Light Scattering.* Springfield, Ill, Thomas, 1973, pp 19, 82

3. Havener WH: *Ocular Pharmacology.* 2d ed. St. Louis, Mosby, 1970, p 12

4. Nesburn AB, Cook ML, Stevens JG: Latent herpes simplex virus: isolation from rabbit trigeminal ganglions between episodes of recurrent infection. Arch Ophthalmol 88:412, 1972

---

*Members of the Jewish faith should, however, be referred to a rabbi in order to confirm that the conditions warrant the donation and that the donation is arranged according to the details of Jewish law.

5. Kibrick S, Takehashi G, Leibowitz HM, et al: Local corticosteroid therapy and reactivation of herpetic keratitis. Arch Ophthalmol 86:694, 1971

6. Litricin MO, Stankoric T: Contributions to the problems of malignant conjunctival tumors of the cornea. Bull Soc Ophtalmol Fr 72:577, 1959

7. Mizuma K: Squamous cell carcinoma of cornea. Arch Ophthalmol 74:807, 1965

8. Radnot M: L'ultrastructures des mastocytes dans les annexes du oculaire. Arch Ophtalmol (Paris) 32:303, 1972

9. Cogan DC, Kinsey VE: Action spectrum of keratitis produced by ultraviolet radiation. Arch Ophthalmol 35:760, 1946

10. Kinsey VE: Spectral transmission of the eye to ultraviolet radiations. Arch Ophthalmol 39:508, 1948

11. Wier KA, Fukuyama K, Epstein WL: Nuclear changes during ultraviolet light-induced depression of ribonucleic acid and protein synthesis in human epidermis. Lab Invest 25:451, 1971

12. Buschke W, Friedenwald JS, Moses SG: Effect of ultraviolet irradiation on corneal epithelium: mitosis, nuclear fragmentation, posttraumatic cell movements, loss of tissue cohesion. J Cell Comp Physiol 26:147, 1945

13. Mishima S: Corneal thickness. Surv Ophthalmol 12:57, 1968

14. Sjögren H, Bloch K: Keratoconjunctivitis sicca and the Sjögren syndrome. Surv Ophthalmol 16:145, 1971

15. Holly FJ, Lemp MA: Wettability and wetting of corneal epithelium. Exp Eye Res 11:239, 1971

16. Baum JL: Systemic disease associated with tear deficiencies. The preocular tear film and dry eye syndromes. Int Ophthalmol Clin 13:170, 1973

17. Coulumbre AJ, Coulumbre JL: The role of intraocular pressure in the development of the chick eye. IV. Corneal curvature. Arch Ophthalmol 59:502, 1958

18. Lancon J, Miller D: Corneal hydration, visual acuity and glare sensitivity. Arch Ophthalmol 90:227, 1973

19. Fresceschetti A: Keratoconus. In: The Cornea. World Congress of the Cornea. Edited by JH King, JW McTigne. Washington, DC, Butterworth, 1965, pp 159–161

20. Rahi A, Davies P, Ruben M, et al: Keratoconus and coexisting atopic disease. Br J Ophthalmol 61:761, 1977

21. Applemans M, Michiels J, Nelis J, et al: Keratoca aiguchez el mongolide. Bull Soc Belge Ophtalmol 128:249, 1961

22. Chi HH, Katzin HM, Teng CC: Histopathology of keratoconus. Am J Ophthalmol 42:847, 1956

23. Schwarz W, Graf Keyselingk D: Electron microscopy of normal and opaque human cornea. In: *The Cornea, Micromolecular Organization of Connective Tissue.* Edited by M Langham. Baltimore, Johns Hopkins Press, 1969, p 123

24. Cogan DG, Albright F, Bartter FC: Hypercalcemia and band keratopathy. Report of nineteen cases. Arch Ophthalmol 40:624, 1948

25. Mapstone P: Normal thermal patterns in cornea and periorbital skin. Br J Ophthalmol 52:818, 1968

26. Slansky HH, Kuwabara T: Intranuclear clear urate crystals in corneal epithelium. Arch Ophthalmol 80:338, 1968

27. Hogan MF, Zimmerman LE: *Ophthalmic Pathology: An Atlas and Textbook.* Philadelphia, Saunders, 1962, p 333

28. Francois J, Feher J: Arcus senilis. Doc Ophthalmol 34:165, 1973

29. Cogan DG, Kuwabara T, Kinoshita J, et al: Ocular manifestations of systemic cystinosis. Arch Ophthalmol 55:36–41, 1956

30. Donaldson D: *Atlas of External Diseases of the Eye,* Vol III. *Cornea and Sclera.* St. Louis, Mosby, 1971, p 74

31. Dikstein S, Maurice DM: The metabolic basis of the fluid pump in the cornea. J Physiol 221:29, 1972

32. Tervo T, Polkama A: Histochemical findings on the Na-K-ATPase activity of the cornea. Acta Ophthalmol (Kbh) 52:88, 1974

33. Fuchs E: Dystrophia epithelialis cornea. Arch Ophthalmol 76:478, 1910

34. Hogan JJ, Wood I, Fine M: Fuchs' endothelial dystrophy of the cornea. 29th Stanford Gifford Memorial Lecture, Am J Ophthalmol 78:363, 1974

35. Inomata H, Smelser GK: Fine structural alterations of corneal endothelium during experimental uveitis. Invest Ophthalmol 9:272, 1970

36. Zirm E: Eine erfolgreiche total Keratoplastick. Albrecht V, Graefes Arch Ophthalmol 64:580, 1906

37. Forster RK, Fine M: The relation of donor age to success in penetrating keratoplasty. Arch Ophthalmol 85:42, 1971

38. Moore TE, Aronson SB: The corneal graft: a multiple variable analysis of the penetrating keratoplasty. Am J Ophthalmol 72:205, 1971

39. Elliott JH: Immune factors in corneal graft rejection. Invest Ophthalmol 10:216, 1971

Chapter 8

Cataract

One of our patients, Mr. Walters, had worked in a camera store for many years before retiring at age 65, after which he spent most of his time reading and visiting his grandchildren in the next town. But about two years after his retirement he had to give up driving at night because oncoming headlights completely blotted out the view of the road, and the tail lights of the cars in front of him were not round, but had a sunburst pattern. Driving into the sun in late afternoon was also difficult because the glare obliterated the road signs. And reading the paper became frustrating. Except for the headlines, it was much easier to ask his wife to read an article aloud. Although during the two years of his retirement Mr. Walters had his glasses changed three times, and even though each change helped a little, his vision seemed to be getting progressively smokier. Nevertheless, he would not admit that his sight was failing; he could, after all, read with the help of that magnifying glass he used for his coin collection.

Mr. Walters's story is typical of a patient who is developing cataracts.

When the lens of the eye becomes cloudy, a patient like Mr. Walters sees the world as if he were looking through a waterfall (Fig. 8-1). At this point he is said to have a cataract (Greek for "waterfall"). Technically, a cataract is not a film or membrane that grows over the eye, but a slow opacification of the lens. The opacification is not caused by the development of scar tissue within the lens, but by molecular rearrangement of the lens components that increases light-scattering. Some cataracts also develop a yellow-brown color due to pigment deposition, which also contributes to this process of opacification.

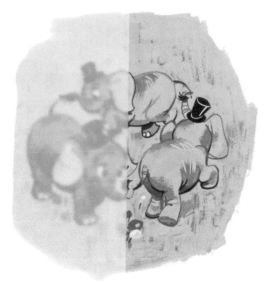

Figure 8-1. Blurred vision caused by cataract *(left)* versus normal vision *(right)*. (Reprinted with permission from *Today Cataract Care.* 56-1270-1. Bausch & Lomb, Soflens Div., Rochester, New York.)

Related Conditions

Although the cause of cataract formation is not known, a number of laboratory findings and clinical associations are helping to fill in the puzzle. Cataracts are more common in diabetic patients than in their normal counterparts. Laboratory experiments have shown that elevated glucose levels in the blood ultimately lead to elevated glucose levels in the lens. Glucose is converted to the sugar alcohol, sorbitol, which *cannot* diffuse out of the lens. *Sorbitol,* a strong osmotic agent, then pulls excess aqueous into the lens, which disrupts the normally transparent arrangement and leads to opacification.[1] Cataracts are also associated with exposure to high doses of x-radiation to the eye, with severe trauma to the eye, and with prolonged episodes of severe inflammation of the ciliary body. Each of these conditions can disrupt the normal function of the lens epithelium.

Laboratory experiments have shown that the lens epithelium has a Na-K-ATPase metabolic pump that removes excess fluid from the lens.[2] These experiments also show that mild trauma or an unphysiologic ionic environment can disturb the metabolic pump and lead to excess fluid build-up in the lens and then to cataract formation. Finally, clinical experience teaches us that prolonged, high-dosage corticosteroid therapy, as prescribed for chronic asthma and/or severe arthritis, leads to the development of cataracts. Laboratory work has demonstrated this by showing that corticosteroids inhibit the metabolic pump of the lens, producing cataracts.[3]

All of these examples have shown that excess fluid within the lens can lead to opacification of the lens. Laboratory investigation has revealed that in cataracts, as opposed to clear lenses, giant molecules of about 50×10^6 molecular weight are responsible for the increased light-scattering.[4] We must now wait to find out how the increased fluid content of the lens influences the production of these giant molecular scatterers.

Types of Cataracts

Cataract development is a slow process that often takes many years. The *posterior subcapsular cataract* is an exception, usually taking less than 24 months to rob the patient of his vision.

Senile cataracts often take ten years or longer to progress to the point of visual incapacity. This variety is divided into three basic groups: the cortical cataract, the nuclear cataract, and a combination of these. In *cortical cataracts,* water-filled clefts open between the lens fibers, creating large differences in refractive index and leading to increased light-scattering. In *nuclear cataracts,* cellular protein forms large, dense aggregates, and a yellow-brown discoloration develops, absorbing and scattering light rays before they reach the retina.

Hypermature cataracts are primarily senile cataracts which have completely opacified. When this happens, the lens cortex begins to liquefy, and the nucleus drops to the bottom of the capsule. Such cataracts tend to leak lens proteins into the anterior chamber, inducing anterior uveitis.

Although most cataracts occur in the elderly, *congenital cataracts* occur in 0.01% of the Western world's juvenile population. The incidence of such cataracts is much greater in the more remote parts of the world, where intermarriage between family members is more frequent. Such inbreeding greatly multiplies the likelihood of birth defects. Of children with such cataracts, one-half will also have other ocular abnormalities, and about one-third will have such other systemic aberrations as convulsions, mental retardation, or hearing problems.

Congenital cataracts can have several causes. If the mother develops certain infections (i.e., rubella, mumps, toxoplasmosis, or syphilis) during the first two months of pregnancy, the infective agent may invade the lens and produce an opacity. About one-third of all patients with congenital cataracts inherit the gene for imperfect lens development from a parent. A significant number of babies born with congenital cataracts have a generalized deficiency of an enzyme that is needed by many tissues (as occurs in galactosemia, aminoaciduria, Down's syndrome, and atopic eczema).

The surgical treatment of congenital cataract differs from that of senile cataracts. In the child, the lens capsule is firmly attached to the vitreous, which has more "body" than that in the elderly patient. The child's vitreous, in turn, has firm attachments to the retina, just as in the adult, and so complete surgical removal of the lens in its capsule could indirectly tear a section of retina and lead to retinal detachment. Therefore, some form of extracapsular approach is used in which the front of the lens is incised and the opaque material aspirated, leaving the rear capsule and its vitreal connections intact.

Numerous types of injuries can cause traumatic cataract. A blow to the eye, if strong enough, may damage the structure of the lens by a shock-wave mechanism. A penetrating injury to the eye from a pencil, for example, may rip open the lens capsule and destroy the lens's clarity. Overexposure to x-rays or gamma-radiation may destroy lens cells and produce an opacity. Once produced, a traumatic cataract will not improve, and surgical removal of the cataract is the only treatment available.

Finally, diabetics run a much greater risk of developing cataracts than do their nondiabetic counterparts. The rate for diabetics is 4 to 6 times greater than that for the population as a whole, and diabetes is the major cause of cataract in patients between the ages of 14 and 44.

History of Therapy

Cataract surgery was apparently developed about 3,000 years ago in India, by a physician named Susruta. In an operation known as "couching," he would puncture the cornea with a special ball-tipped knife. He then punched the cataractous lens backward so that it dropped into the vitreous out of the patient's line of sight. The operation was done without anesthesia, the coucher sitting in front of the patient.[5] The maneuver took less than a minute, and the instantaneous results were impressive, for the patient was taken from blindness to usable vision. The wise coucher then collected his fee and left the village while the patient was pleased, for the satisfaction was usually short-lived. If the lens was not pushed into the vitreous perfectly, a severe inflammation of the eye would soon ensue, and the patient would be left with a painful, blind eye. Couching, though illegal, is still performed in the back-country villages of India.

Interestingly, a form of couching has been resurrected recently in the People's Republic of China, where there are far many more patients than that country's small number of ophthalmologists can treat. Chinese "barefoot doctors" now do a partial couching, in which the superior zonules are broken and the cataract, still hinged to the ciliary processes by the inferior zonules, is pushed back into the vitreous. The technique involves a very small incision and no suturing, thus requiring a very short hospital stay and allowing the patient a speedy return to work.

The first successful attempt in cataract surgery, as we practice it today, was made by Jacques Daviel in 1756. The patient was a young painter whose cataracts had cost him his sight. He sought out Dr. Daviel and stated that he would risk everything to see again. During the surgery, the cornea was opened at the limbus and the lens was noted to be quite firm. Daviel loosened the lens from its anatomic moorings, cut a portion of the iris out of the way, and pushed the cataract out of the eye with a blunt spatula. No sutures were used to close the wound. By the twentieth postoperative day the patient, with the use of spectacles, got around without difficulty. In 1866 Henry Williard Williams, a graduate of Harvard Medical School, successfully used a suture to close the wound after a cataract was removed.[6] Sutureless cataract surgery is still performed in certain backwoods parts of the world today. Although in most instances the unsutured eye seals itself properly, modern sutures guarantee proper wound alignment in almost all cases.

Modern Treatment

Surgery

Today, cataract extraction is performed under local or general anesthesia, and the operation lasts less than an hour. An incision of about 180° is made along the outer border of the cornea (limbal incision, Fig. 8-2). The surgeon injects α-chymotrypsin (a proteolytic enzyme) into the eye to dissolve the ligaments that hold the lens in place; he then removes the lens intact (*intracapsular extraction,* Fig. 8-3), and sutures the wound (Fig. 8-2). At the surgeon's discretion, sutures are either left in place or removed in a few weeks.

The cataract operation may also be performed as an *extracapsular extraction.* After entry into the anterior chamber, the surgeon makes an opening in the transparent lens capsule. The surgeon then aspirates the cloudy cataractous material from the lens, leaving the clear capsule still anchored by zonules and thus keeping the vitreous body in its normal position. Earlier in the century, the extracapsular extraction was the most popular form of cataract surgery. Since aspiration of the lens contents was easier when the substance of the lens was completely soft and opaque (mature cataract), the surgeon would often tell the patient to wait for surgery until the cataract was ripe. Because of present-day surgical instrumentation, the patient need not wait for the cataract to ripen in order to undergo successful surgery.

A recent variant of the conventional operation involves the use of a miniature combination grinder, aspirator, and irrigator. This tiny device *(phacoemulsifier)* is placed into the eye through a small incision, the capsule is opened, the lens interior is ground and mixed with water, and the

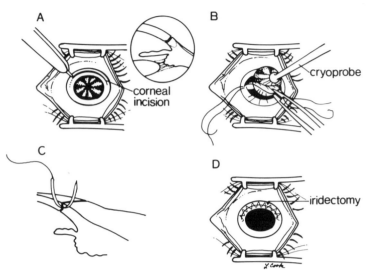

Figure 8-2. The major steps in cataract surgery. **A** Limbal incision. **B** Removal of cataract (see Fig. 8-3). **C** Corneal suture at close of surgery. **D** Appearance of sutures under conjunctival flap.

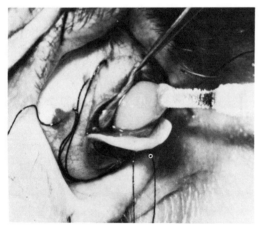

Figure 8-3. Removal of a cataractous lens with a cryo-applicator.

resulting suspension is aspirated from the eye. This extracapsular extraction seems to work better in the younger patient whose cataract has not hardened excessively, and thus is more easily debrided (Fig. 8-4). With either type of procedure the patient is usually up and around on the day of surgery and leaves the hospital within a few days. Normal physical activity is resumed in a month or two.

Naturally, the approach to surgery must meet the social and economic needs of the country. Whereas China has used their barefoot

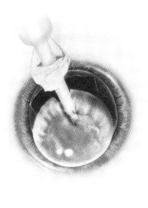

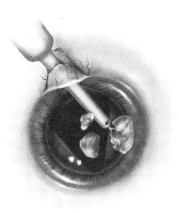

Figure 8-4. Photograph of phacoemulsifier at work. *Top:* The tip of the handpiece begins breaking up and aspirating the cataract. *Bottom:* A few fragments remain. Note the clear pupil. (Reprinted with permission from Cavitron Surgical Corporation, Div. of Syntel Inc., Irvine, California.)

doctors and a modified couching technique, India has organized weekend cataract camps in rural areas. A thousand patients or more attend an outdoor camp in which their cataracts are removed by a team of volunteer ophthalmic surgeons and nursing personnel. Anesthesia for each operation depends on a few drops of cocaine instilled into the eye preoperatively and on the patient's cooperation. The surgical approach is the conventional intracapsular extraction. If the patient moves, the doctor slaps the patient's face as a reminder to stay still. Occasionally, the significance of such a slap is misinterpreted. The story is told that at the close of one of these weekend camps, one of the operated patients ran up to one of the surgeons and asked him to slap the other side of his face.

"Why?" asked the doctor. "Because I have a cataract growing in that eye also."

No medical treatment can dissolve cataracts or prevent their development; surgery is the *only* therapy currently available. Surgical intervention is recommended when the cataract interferes with the patient's way of life. While a patient whose livelihood depends on his ability to see fine detail will need surgery when the cataract is still small, others may not need to undergo surgery until their cataract is more advanced.

Since the lens is removed in cataract surgery, its focusing power must be replaced with spectacles or with a contact lens (see below). Since such replacement may cause a problem when a cataract occurs in only one eye and vision in the other eye is clear, surgery in this case is recommended only in the following circumstances: (1) if the hazy vision in the eye with the cataract interferes with vision in the good eye; (2) if the cataract is mature, i.e., totally opaque (such a cataract usually degenerates into a milky, liquid—hypermature—cataract that is difficult to remove by intracapsular extraction); (3) if the patient has a significant cataract developing in the second eye as well. In the latter instance, it is best to complete treatment of the first eye, so that the patient can use this eye when the other eye is to be operated on and then bandaged.

Optical Correction of Aphakia

Because the lens is removed at surgery, a new optical system is needed to focus the outside world into the retina. Traditionally, thick, high-powered spectacles have been used. Although effective, they magnify and distort everything the patient looks at. Anyone familiar with a magnifying glass, for instance, knows that the farther the glass is moved from the object under scrutiny, the greater the magnification. In correcting an aphakic patient, the farther the correcting element is from the retina, the greater the magnification. Thus aphakic spectacles magnify more than contact lenses, and contact lenses magnify a bit more than intraocular lenses. The aphakic patient fitted with the traditional glasses therefore requires a high degree of adaptive power to return to an active life (Fig. 8-5).

Special contact lenses have been a major advance for the aphakic patient. With a contact lens, things look almost as they did before the cataract developed. Unfortunately, the lenses available at present must be removed every evening and inserted in the morning, and this task proves to be too difficult for many elderly people (Fig. 8-6).

Appreciating the optical problems following cataract surgery, surgeons have been experimenting since 1950 with a plastic lens that is left in the eye after the cataract is removed. Within the past 25 years, many of the original problems connected with artificial lens implantation have been solved, and the intraocular plastic lens is much improved. Because the lenses are often held in the proper position by interdigitating with the

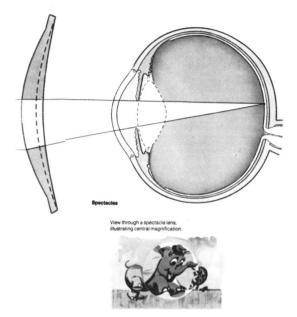

Spectacles

View through a spectacle lens,
illustrating central magnification.

Figure 8-5. Magnified appearance of the elephant as seen with aphakic spectacles. (Reprinted with permission from *Today Cataract Care*. 56-1270-1. Bausch & Lomb, Soflens Div., Rochester, New York.)

iris and pupil, the nonophthalmologist should not dilate the pupil of an eye with an intraocular lens without checking with the ophthalmologist first.

Some surgeons use these intraocular lenses routinely. The problems currently preventing wider acceptance include increased corneal trauma during lens insertion, possible dislocation of the lens after surgery, and interference with full visualization of the peripheral retina by the ophthalmologist. Because there is a 2% incidence of retinal detachment following all cataract surgery, interference with visualization of peripheral retinal detachments can frustrate proper diagnosis and treatment of this problem (Fig. 8-7).

Scientists are, however, close to perfecting a continuous-wear aphakic contact lens. Such a lens, when ready, will transmit freely all of the gases and nutrients needed for corneal health, will not accumulate secretions or dry out, and will be worn for months at a time. It is expected that such a lens will be ready in the near future.

Surgical Prognosis

If the cataract extraction has been done properly from a technical standpoint, and if the structures of the eye were healthy before surgery, the patient's sight will be better postoperatively in 90% to 95% of such

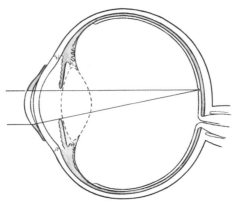

Figure 8-6. Optics of an aphakic contact lens. (Reprinted with permission from *Today Cataract Care.* 56-1270-1. Bausch & Lomb, Soflens Div., Rochester, New York.)

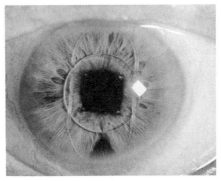

Figure 8-7. Postoperative photograph of an intraocular lens in place.

cases. The trauma inherent in the operation will, however, lead to the following complications in a small percentage of subjects.

Cystoid Macular Edema. In some unknown way, about 50% of those patients who undergo surgery develop an accumulation of fluid within the macula and a subsequent drop in visual acuity one to three months after surgery.[7] This condition will slowly repair itself, so that usually within months only about 5% of the original group will still have macular edema.[8]

Corneal Edema. Cataract surgery injures or destroys about 10% of the corneal endothelial cells.[9] In those patients with low preoperative endothelial cell counts, a loss of another 10% may lead to corneal decompensation, excess fluid accumulation within the cornea, increased corneal light-scattering, and, ultimately, diminished corneal clarity. About 1% of all cataract surgery is followed by this condition, known as *aphakic bullous keratopathy*.[10] Operations involving intraocular lens implantation or phacoemulsification may further traumatize the corneal endothelium, and so these patients are more likely to develop bullous keratopathy in the ensuing years.

Retinal Detachment. It is felt that the forward movement of the vitreous after the cataract is removed may tear the retina and ultimately detach it in about 2% of those operated on. Patients most prone to postoperative retinal detachment include patients with thin or diseased areas of retina.[11]

Glaucoma. In some patients, eye-rubbing or forceful coughing and sneezing may lead to a small wound leak soon after surgery. This complication may produce a flat anterior chamber and, ultimately, *pupillary-block glaucoma.* Pupillary-block glaucoma may also be the result of a severe inflammatory response to the surgery *(postoperative iridocyclitis).* If not treated vigorously, adhesions between the vitreous face and the iris develop, resulting in angle-closure glaucoma. Most cases of postoperative glaucoma are treatable, but a fraction of 1% of those patients undergoing cataract extraction develop an uncontrollable glaucoma that results in blindness.

Other Complications. A host of extremely rare but devastating complications of cataract surgery, such as intraocular infection or hemorrhage, are mentioned in most textbooks. Undue emphasis on these complications tends to obscure the point that cataract surgery has a better prognosis than almost any other operation done today.

References

1. Varma SD, Kinoshita JH: Sorbitol pathway in diabetic and galactosemic rat lens. Biochim Biophys Acta 338:632, 1974

2. Palva M, Palkama A: Electron microscopical, histochemical and biochemical findings on the Na-K-ATPase activity in the epithelium of rat lens. Exp Eye Res 22:229, 1976

3. Mayman CI, Miller D, Tijerina ML: In vitro formation of steroid cataract in bovine lens. Invest Ophthalmol Visual Sci [Suppl] 17:234, 1978

4. Jedziniak JA, Kinoshita JH, Yates EM, Hocker LO, Benedek GB: On the presence and mechanism of formation of heavy molecular weight aggregates in human normal and cataractous lenses. Exp Eye Res 15:185, 1973

5. Bellows JG: *Cataract and Anomalies of the Lens.* St. Louis, Mosby, 1944, pp 19, 422

6. Snyder C: *Our Ophthalmic Heritage.* Boston, Little Brown, 1967, p 41

7. Hitchings RA, Chisholm IH, Bird AC: Aphakic macular edema. Incidence and pathogenesis. Invest Ophthalmol 14:68, 1975

8. Hitchings RA: Aphakic macular edema: a two-year follow-up study. Br J Ophthalmol 61:628, 1977

9. Sugar J, Mitchelson J, Kraff M: The effect of phacoemulsification on corneal endothelial cell density. Arch Ophthalmol 96:446, 1978

10. Jaffee NS: *Cataract Surgery and its Complications,* 2d ed. St. Louis, Mosby, 1972, p 191

11. Norton EWD: Retinal detachment in aphakia. Am J Ophthalmol 58:111, 1964

Chapter 9

Glaucoma

I was called to the emergency room late one night to help treat an elderly couple. Mr. Coleman, a man of 70, had awakened that night with chest pains and trouble breathing. He had suffered a myocardial infarction and was rushed to the intensive care unit. Mrs. Coleman, an apprehensive lady of 65, had attempted to make her husband more comfortable, when all at once she noted pain in her eyes and an inability to see clearly. Upon interview, Mrs. Coleman reported nausea and pain in both eyes, and she could see me only as a vague outline. When she looked at my examining light, she told me that she saw many colored rings surrounding it. Her visual acuity was counting fingers at two feet, her corneas looked steamy, her eyes quite red, her pupils large, and the reading on the tonometer was 80 mmHg, O.U. "Clearly a case of angle-closure glaucoma," said the young intern. "Mrs. Coleman should be admitted to the hospital, treated medically until the intraocular pressure returns to normal, and then have bilateral peripheral iridectomies performed." He was right.

Causes

Glaucoma may be of either the *angle-closure* or *open-angle* type.[1] Acute angle-closure glaucoma (Fig. 9-1) may develop in an eye whose angle is already narrow and becomes narrower as the lens accumulates fibers and thickens with age, slowly pushing the iris forward. The filtration angle can be closed if the pupil becomes so widely dilated that it is brought into contact with the midperiphery of the lens. The iris then becomes jammed against the lens and locks the aqueous out of the anterior chamber. As pressure builds up within the posterior chamber, the iris balloons

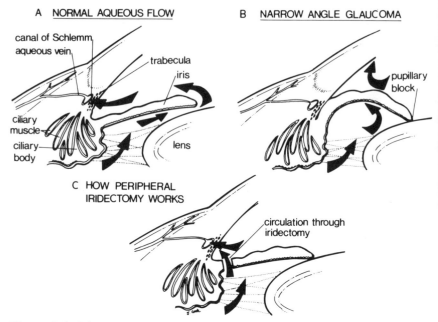

A NORMAL AQUEOUS FLOW

canal of Schlemm,
aqueous vein,
trabecula
iris
ciliary
muscle
ciliary
body
lens

B NARROW ANGLE GLAUCOMA

pupillary
block

C HOW PERIPHERAL
IRIDECTOMY WORKS

circulation through
iridectomy

Figure 9-1. Diagrams representing **A** normal aqueous flow, **B** an attack of angle-closure glaucoma, and **C** the method by which a peripheral iridectomy breaks the attack of angle-closure glaucoma. (Artist: Laurel Cook.)

forward, obstructing the filtration angle and further contributing to increased intraocular pressure. Attacks of acute angle-closure glaucoma usually involve eye pain, redness, and corneal edema with its attendant blurred vision.

The majority (well over 50%) of patients with glaucoma, however, have the open-angle variety. In these eyes, it is not the iris that occludes the filtration angle, but some submicroscopic defect that prevents aqueous outflow. This condition never causes pain or redness, and the intraocular pressure rises slowly and insidiously.

No chapter on glaucoma would be complete without mention of steroid-induced glaucoma. In 1949, Hench et al.[2] isolated cortisone from the adrenal gland and noted its antiinflammatory properties. In the early 1950s, cortisone eyedrops were introduced, and for a while steroid drops were the panacea whenever eyes were annoyingly inflamed (no matter the cause). In 1962, Goldmann reported a number of patients who developed rapid-onset open-angle glaucoma with visual-field loss.[3] A thorough medical history revealed that the patients had been using cortisone eyedrops for a number of months. We still do not know the mechanism by which steroid eyedrops produce glaucoma, but about one-third of all patients on chronic oral or topical steroid therapy develop elevated intraocular pressures. The condition reverses itself when steroids are discontinued, but if the optic nerve has been damaged by the increased pressure, the damage is usually permanent. The quest continues for a steroid that will quell inflammation without inducing glaucoma.

A relatively rare variety of glaucoma characterized by progressive neofibrovascular changes of the iris *(rubeosis iridis)* and the trabecular meshwork is known as *neovascular glaucoma.* It is associated with proliferative diabetic retinopathy and occlusion of the central or branch retinal vein. In the latter instance, it is called 100-day glaucoma, because if neovascular glaucoma develops, it will occur within 100 days of the venous occlusion. The mechanism of this form of glaucoma is unclear, but appears to be a sequelae of retinal hypoxia.

In *postcontusion glaucoma,* severe trauma to the eye tears the root of the iris from its mooring, tearing along with it the connection of the ciliary muscle to the trabecular meshwork. If the damage is extensive enough, postcontusion or angle recession glaucoma will develop.

The bulk of glaucoma research suggests that the *increased intraocular pressure constricts the capillaries that supply the fibers of the optic nerve.* Acutely elevated pressure over a few days, or chronic mild pressure over 5 to 10 years, destroys the fibers of the optic nerve. The first fibers to die are often those that record the events in the peripheral retina. Central vision is lost later. Once vision is lost, it is rarely restored even if the pressure returns to normal levels. As more nerve substance is lost, cupping of the optic disc increases (see *Diagnosis*). The paleness of the diseased cup is primarily the result of *reactive gliosis,* with capillary closure a secondary mechanism.

Both angle-closure and open-angle glaucoma are rare in infants and children, but together occur in about 2% of the adult population over 40 years of age. Glaucoma may have a hereditary basis; it develops more frequently in those with relatives who have the condition and is also found a bit more frequently in diabetics. Interestingly, glaucoma of any type is rare among Melanesians, Polynesians, Mongolians, and Bedouins. Angle-closure glaucoma is more common among the people of Thailand, Vietnam, Burma, Java, and Europe. Open-angle glaucoma is more common in Scandinavia and the United States.[4]

Diagnosis

Since open-angle glaucoma can develop insidiously, and because damage from elevated intraocular pressure is preventable, routine tonometry in people over 40 is important. The average intraocular pressure in the healthy adult population is 15 mmHg. A tension greater than 22 mmHg is highly suspicious and should be evaluated more completely by an ophthalmologist.

Examination of the optic nerve with the ophthalmoscope is also important in detecting glaucoma and following its progress. Within the optic disc is a physiologic cup (Fig. 9-2). The white base of the cup is the

A   B

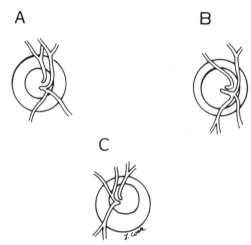

C

Figure 9-2. Drawings illustrating variations in cup:disc ratio in normal patients. **A** The cup:disc ratio is about 0.4, but the cup is round and the blood vessels emerge from the center of the disc. **B** The disc is larger and the cup:disc ratio is about 0.6, but the cup is round and the blood vessels emerge from the center of the disc. **C** The disc is slightly tilted, producing an eccentric cup, with the blood vessels again emerging from the center of the disc. (Artist: Laurel Cook.)

visible part of the *lamina cribrosa,* the area of the sclera that is sievelike in structure to accommodate passage of the optic-nerve fibers out of the eye. The normal mottled pattern of the lamina cribrosa is visible where there are few nerve fibers, which occupy the rim of the optic disc. The normal rim appears pink in relation to the cup because of the presence of blood vessels, which nourish the nerve fibers. The ratio of the diameter of the cup to the overall diameter of the disc is 0.3 or less in about 70% of the population.[5]

What should you do if you discover that the cup:disc ratio is greater than the normal 0.3? Such an optic nerve is probably more vulnerable to increased intraocular pressure or already shows signs of glaucomatous damage. Other features of the disc should be evaluated. Is the cup symmetric or is its vertical extent greater than the horizontal (Fig. 9-3)? Greater vertical extent suggests glaucomatous change. Is the cup the same in each eye? Asymmetry suggests glaucoma. Are the cup depressions deep or shallow? Deeper cups are caused by progressing glaucoma. After such analysis, perform tonometry. If the pressure is over 22 mmHg, the physician should suspect glaucoma. If the pressure is below 22 mmHg, the patient's pressure should be checked yearly.

Suppose that the cup:disc ratio is small (0.2), but that the pressure is 25 mmHg. Such an optic nerve has an efficient blood supply and will probably be able to tolerate this pressure without damage. In this case, the ophthalmologist may elect to forgo immediate medical treatment and, instead, to follow the patient by taking periodic photographs of the disc.

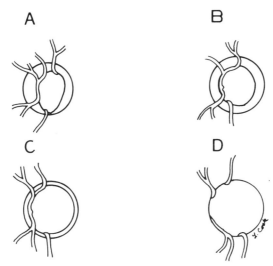

A

B

C

D

Figure 9-3. Four stages of glaucomatous discs. **A** The cup:disc ratio is 0.5, the cup is enlarged vertically, and the blood vessels appear to originate deep in the floor of the cup and to curl around the edge as they emerge. **B** The cup:disc ratio is 0.6, the cup appears deep, and the blood vessels have all been pushed toward the nose. **C** The cup:disc ratio is 0.8, the cup is very deep, the blood vessels are pushed toward the nose and curl up onto the retinal level as if from a deep excavation. **D** The disc is totally cupped; this eye would be completely blind. (Artist: Laurel Cook.)

Although the cup:disc ratio is valuable in estimating progressive disc damage, it is not infallible. In glaucoma, the cup:disc ratio usually gives us a sense of functioning neuroretinal tissue, but if a disc is 1 mm in diameter and has no cup, it will have the same number of nerve fibers as a congenitally large disc of 1.1 mm diameter that has a cup:disc ratio of 0.4. Thus, a patient with a congenitally large optic disc and a high cup:disc ratio may appear to have glaucomatous damage, but may in fact be normal.[5] Thus, the concept of cup:disc ratio determining disc vulnerability to elevated intraocular pressure is useful but not perfect.

The visual field test is probably the most accurate method of demonstrating nerve fiber damage due to glaucoma. The test is very important in charting progress in advanced glaucoma, where the disc is no longer capable of showing subtle deterioration in color, cup depth, or cup:disc ratio.[6] Figures 9-4 and 9-5 show typical early changes in the visual field *(Bjerrum scotoma)* of the glaucoma patient.

Treatment

A diagnosis of glaucoma terrifies many patients who assume that it means ultimate blindness no matter what treatment is instituted. Therefore, a

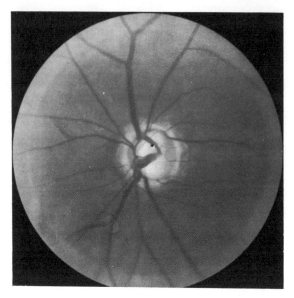

Figure 9-4. Photograph of a glaucomatous disc. The cup:disc ratio is 0.6, the disc is elongated vertically with almost no vertical rim of neural tissue, and the vessels are pushed toward the nose, curling around the edge of the disc.

crucial part of treatment is to impart the message that the patient was fortunate to have his or her glaucoma discovered early, because proper treatment can prevent loss of sight. This is also true in the case of an attack of angle-closure glaucoma; if medication or surgery lowers the pressure sufficiently in less than 24–48 hours, little or no vision will be lost. The salient criteria that determine the degree of damage are the degree of intraocular pressure increase, the vulnerability of the optic nerve to compression (often, the larger the cup, the higher the vulnerability), and the duration of pressure elevation.

Acute Angle-Closure Glaucoma

An attack of acute angle-closure glaucoma is an emergency situation. Once the diagnosis is established, the patient must be hospitalized. Drops (such as pilocarpine) are instilled into the eye every 15 minutes to constrict the pupil, to pull the iris away from the lens, and to allow the iris to move out of the angle. Such a program may relieve the attack. In some cases, however, the iris becomes paralyzed by the prolonged increased pressure, requiring other measures to lower the pressure. Such systemic medications as carbonic-anhydrase inhibitors, which diminish the production of aqueous, and hyperosmotic agents (e.g., glycerol, mannitol, or urea), which draw fluid out of the eye, may be administered. Once the intraocular pressure has been lowered by these agents, pilocarpine is again effective. When the pressure returns to normal, the patient is

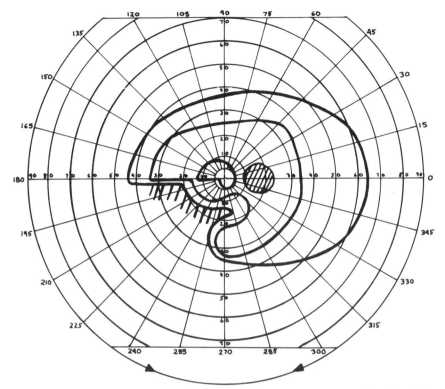

Figure 9-5. The visual field of the patient in Figure 9-4. The visual-field loss is in the inferior nasal quadrant. (Artist: Laurel Cook.)

prepared for surgery. A peripheral *iridectomy* (Fig. 9-6) is performed in which a small hole is made in the iris to prevent build-up of pressure behind the iris and, thus, to prevent closure of the angle. Postoperatively, most of these patients need no further medications.

Chronic Open-Angle Glaucoma

Medication. Most patients with open-angle glaucoma must take medication for the rest of their lives. Three types of medication are currently in use.

Miotics constrict the pupil (the circular ciliary-muscle fibers) and open the drainage pores in the angle. This group of medications include such parasympathomimetic agents as *pilocarpine, echothiophate iodide* (Phospholine Iodide®), and *carbachol.* The patient must use these drops for the rest of his life, two to four times daily. A recent development is the Occusert®, a small, soft-plastic conjunctival insert that is worn under the lower lid. Impregnated with pilocarpine, it allows the drug to diffuse into the eye at a slow, even rate over the course of a week and is then replaced. This slow

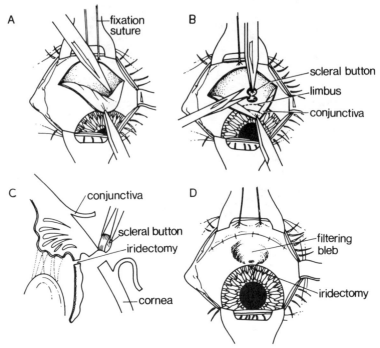

Figure 9-6. The steps in one kind of filtering operation. **A** Dissection of conjunctival flap. **B** Removal of scleral button. **C** Cross-sectional view of removal of scleral button and iridectomy. **D** Postoperative appearance of eye. (Artist: Laurel Cook.)

diffusion eliminates the temporary blurring of vision associated with the use of conventional pilocarpine drops. Miotics effectively control the intraocular pressure, but have a major drawback: the small pupil that results from their use increases the visual handicap in a patient with developing cataracts. The combination of a constricted pupil and cataract makes the world even more dim.

Epinephrine eyedrops diminish the production of aqueous humor. Since they dilate the pupil only slightly, they do not produce the visual discomfort caused by miotics. Unhappily, epinephrine (a vasoconstrictor), if used regularly, can induce a rebound dilation of the conjunctival vessels and make the eyes appear chronically red. Epinephrine is often used in conjunction with pilocarpine.

Secretion of aqueous humor by the ciliary body depends on two factors: the presence of the enzyme carbonic anhydrase and a neutral pH. If a carbonic-anhydrase inhibitor such as acetazolamide is taken by mouth, the secretion of aqueous is decreased and the pressure in the eye goes down. Unfortunately, some patients are sensitive to this medication, and its use is limited by unpleasant side effects (e.g., gastrointestinal disturbance, generalized weakness, and a disturbing tingling of the fingers).

Recently, β-adrenergic blocking agents have been shown to help lower intraocular pressure in glaucoma. The mechanism of action probably involves a decrease in the secretion of aqueous.[7]

Surgery. If medication fails to lower the elevated intraocular pressure or if the patient refuses to take the proper medication, surgery must be considered. There are two surgical approaches: improve the drainage or decrease secretion of aqueous.

Customarily, the first approach (called a *filtering procedure*) improves drainage by making a hole in the sclera (Fig. 9-6). Subsequently, the aqueous flows through this hole, collecting in a filtering bleb under the conjunctiva. Some feel that the blood vessels in the conjunctiva overlying the bleb continually absorb the excess aqueous, but this process is not completely understood. The operation is successful in a majority of cases. Failure is usually due to an overgrowth of fibrous tissue, which plugs the surgical hole. This complication is quite common in black patients. Other forms of filtering procedures, called *trabeculectomies* and *sinusotomies,* involve making finer, more localized openings.

If filtering surgery fails, an attempt is made to destroy part of the ciliary body in order to partially shut off the production of aqueous. This can be accomplished by freezing the ciliary body with a cryoprobe, applying the instrument to the outside of the eye directly over portions of the ciliary body.

References

1. Chandler PA, Grant WM: *Lectures on Glaucoma.* Philadelphia, Lea & Febiger, 1965, pp 1–100

2. Hench PS, Kendall EC, Slocumb CH, et al: The effect of a hormone of the adrenal cortex (17-hydroxy-11-dehydrocorticosterone; compound E) and pituitary adrenocorticotropic hormone in rheumatoid arthritis. Proc Staff Meet Mayo Clin 24:181, 1949

3. Goldmann H: Cortisone glaucoma. Arch Ophthalmol 68:621, 1962

4. Fuchs A: *Geography of Eye Diseases.* Vienna, Verley der Wissenschaftlichen Verbade, 1962, pp 65–71

5. Drance SM: The disc and the field in glaucoma. Trans Am Acad Ophthalmol Otolaryngol 85:209, 1978

6. Hitchings RA, Spaeth GL: The optic disc in glaucoma. II. Correlation of the appearance of the optic disc with the visual field. Br J Ophthalmol 61:107, 1977

7. Yablonski ME, Zimmerman TJ, Waltman SR, et al: A fluorophotometric study of the effect of topical timolol on aqueous humor dynamics. Paper presented at ARVO, Sarasota, Florida, 1978

Chapter 10

Strabismus

In any discussion of the precision of vocabulary, one is reminded of the story of how Senator George Smathers once campaigned against his opponent Claude Pepper. "Are you aware," Smathers would say, "that Claude Pepper is known all over Washington as a shameless extrovert? Not only that, but this man is reliably reported to practice nepotism with his sister-in-law, and he has a sister who was once a thespian in wicked New York. Worst of all, it is an established fact that Mr. Pepper, before his marriage, practiced celibacy." The field of strabismus (also called "squint") has a special vocabulary, and although many of its terms sound like familiar words, they are precise and unique. In order to guard against Smathersian abuse and confusion, these terms are defined below:

ALTERNATING STRABISMUS: Either eye may turn, while the fellow eye does the seeing.

AMBLYOPIA: Poor vision without any apparent disease of the eye or refractive error.

CONVERGENCE: The process of directing the visual axes of the two eyes inward.

DIVERGENCE: The process of directing the visual axes of the two eyes outward.

ESOPHORIA: A tendency of either eye to turn in.

ESOTROPIA: The condition in which one eye is often or always turned in (also known as *convergent strabismus* or *crossed eye*).

EXOPHORIA: A tendency of either eye to turn out.

EXOTROPIA: The condition in which one eye is often or always turned out (also known as *divergent strabismus* or *walleye*).

FUSION: The power of coordinating the images received by the two eyes into a single mental image.

HYPERPHORIA: A tendency for either eye to turn up.

HYPERTROPIA: The condition in which one eye turns up.

NEAR POINT OF ACCOMMODATION: The nearest point at which the eye can perceive an object clearly.

NEAR POINT OF CONVERGENCE: The nearest point at which the two eyes can direct their visual axes and maintain fusion.

STEREOPSIS: The ability to perceive the solidity of objects and their relative position in space without such clues as shadow, size, and overlapping.

Types of Strabismus

Twenty percent of all strabismics are *exotropes* and 80% are *esotropes*. The exotropes are divided into those that squint *constantly,* and those who do so only *intermittently* (as, for example, when a child is tired). Most exotropes have *alternating strabismus*; that is, sometimes the right eye turns out and sometimes the left eye turns out.

Esotropes also may be constant or intermittent. But unlike exotropes, most esotropes are constant, and roughly 50% have the alternating variety. Table 10-1 summarizes the types of strabismus by incidence.

Amblyopia is a type of decreased or distorted vision primarily seen in the constantly turned eye of all strabismus patients. Amblyopia is not seen in the alternating-strabismic patient. In some way that is not completely understood, visual information from the turned eye is suppressed in the cerebral cortex. If untreated during a child's formative years, the suppression of vision from one eye becomes a permanent characteristic of the processing center of the brain, and the eye operates as if it were blind or amblyopic.

Table 10-1. Types, Relative Incidences, and Characteristics of Strabismus

Type	Percentage of All Strabismus	Constant vs. Intermittent	Alternating vs. Nonalternating
Exotropia	20%	Most intermittent	Most alternating
Esotropia	80%	Most constant	50%/50%

Patients may be amblyopic for reasons other than strabismus, and the reader is advised to reread the case discussed in Chapter 1.

Causes

Getting both eyes to look at the same object at the same time is a very complicated task that requires good vision in each eye, smooth functioning of the coordinating centers of the brain, and normal extraocular muscles. Surprisingly, in spite of all these requirements, most people have straight eyes and only about 2% to 3% have strabismus.

Ocular Influence

In *congenital toxoplasmosis* (an infection produced by the intracellular sporozoan parasite *Toxoplasma gondii*), the retinal fovea of one of the eyes is often attacked by the parasite and destroyed, thus reducing central vision in that eye. Fifty percent of those patients with toxoplasmatic destruction of the fovea have esotropia.

There is a higher-than-normal incidence of strabismus in children who do not see well out of one eye as a result of congenital cataracts, corneal scars, or a large refractive error in one eye. If either eye in the developing child fails to send a clear signal to the visual part of the brain, inaccurate positioning of the eyes may occur.

Brain Influence

For those with normal vision (emmetropes), the brain coordinates eye movement and lens accommodation so that a target is squarely placed on each fovea and kept in sharp focus. The process of accommodation requires a different program of commands in hyperopia (farsightedness), for the hyperope must accommodate an extra amount to see clearly. Since accommodation and convergence are coupled actions, hyperopes tend to overconverge on a target. In such individuals, the brain's fusion center must compensate so that the eyes maintain proper binocular fixation at all times. These compensating signals override the excess convergence and bring the eyes into alignment. In some hyperopes, the fusion influence is not strong enough to do this, and the extra accommodative convergence causes one eye to turn in. Because of the brain's major role in the maintenance of straight eyes, the incidence of strabismus is higher in patients with altered brain functions.*

---

*Interestingly, recent neurophysiologic experiments on Siamese kittens (many of whom have strabismus) suggest that their nasal retinas overwhelm their temporal retinas in brain representation. Thus, the squinting position is an adaptation to their imbalanced neural

The incidence of esotropia among people with Down's syndrome, for example, is about 50%,[1] and the incidence of strabismus is higher in premature infants and in infants whose mothers suffered from toxemia during pregnancy.[2] Interestingly, almost half of the children who undergo surgery for their squints straighten their eyes as they are being put to sleep with general anesthesia.[3] If no surgery is performed, the eyes return to the strabismic position when the patient awakens. This also suggests that certain areas of the brain may exert excessive influence on eye position in the strabismic patient.

Extraocular Muscle Influence

The anatomic abnormalities present in some extraocular muscles may cause strabismus. In esotropia, for example, the insertion of the *medial rectus muscle* is often too close to the front of the eye, giving that muscle an unfair mechanical advantage. When it contracts, it pulls the eye inward abnormally. Surgeons often report abnormally weak *lateral recti* in cases of esotropia, and unusually thin *medial recti* in some cases of exotropia. Roughly 1% of all cases of squint are caused by an actual paralysis of one of the extraocular muscles.[2]

We do, then, understand the cause of strabismus in some patients, but in most patients the etiology is still a mystery.

History of Treatment

In the mid-1700s, Dr. George L. deBuffon suggested that the presence of an amblyopic eye was the cause of squint. He had placed the cart before the horse, but he rightly recommended occlusion of the good eye. Johann Friederich Dieffenbach of Berlin, who is considered to be the legitimate father of strabismus surgery and who first reported his work in 1839, weakened what he considered an overactive extraocular muscle by cutting its tendon, thus allowing the muscle to snap back and to reattach at a point farther back on the globe. This maneuver diminished the muscle's mechanical advantage and recentered the eye. Later in the nineteenth century, Louis Emile Javal, a French oculist, proposed his theory of fusion deficiency as the cause of squint. At the turn of the century, Javal's work was amplified and extended by Worth, who recommended various orthoptic exercises for deficient fusion.[4]

Since that time, elaborate stereoscopes, sophisticated surgical instruments, and lengthy analyses of the results of treatment have been brought

---

makeup, in an effort to balance the influence of the light falling on the retinas. (Guillery RW, Casagrande VA, Oberdorfer MD: Congenitally abnormal vision in Siamese cats. Nature 252:195, 1974.)

to bear on the problem of strabismus. There have been, however, no conceptual breakthroughs concerning cause or cure during the twentieth century—a regrettable lack in view of the needs of the four million American children (2% of the population) who have squint. Even though our understanding of strabismus is incomplete, however, most strabismic patients can be helped through proper diagnosis and treatment.

Diagnosing Esotropia

The physician should fully determine all of the nuances of the patient's squint (i.e., intermittent, alternating, etc.), because a proper categorization will suggest not only the ideal treatment, but also the chances for both cosmetic and functional cure.

History

Find out the age of onset of the squint. If the age of onset is at birth, or within the first 12 months of age, the prognosis for the development of fusion is very poor.[5,6]

Visual Acuity

It is important to find out if amblyopia is present for two reasons: in general, amblyopia cannot be corrected after age 12,[7] and the prognosis for improvement in fusion is better if the vision in each eye is equal to or better than 20/50.

Cycloplegic Refraction

The 10% to 20% of all esotropia that is caused by overaccommodation may sometimes be corrected with proper glasses. To determine the refractive error when no accommodation is present, the accommodation must be temporarily paralyzed by cycloplegic eyedrops. In about 50% of all cases of esotropia, overaccommodation contributes to the condition, and so spectacles will impart some improvement.

Fusion

The examiner must determine whether both foveas record imagery and coordinate what they see at the same time. In the red-glass test, one means of checking fusion, one eye is covered with a red filter and the patient is asked to look at a white light. The red filter identifies the contribution of that eye while viewing the white light. If a single pink light is seen, both eyes are fusing properly. If separate red and white lights are reported, the patient has diplopia (perception of two images of a single object). If only a red or white light is reported, then vision is suppressed in one eye and there is no fusion.

Extraocular Muscle Function

Testing the function of all the extraocular muscles is important, even though only 1% of all squint is caused by paralysis of a muscle. If the examination reveals that one muscle is paretic, its antagonist muscle should be weakened surgically. Such a finding suggests that other neurologic defects may also be present.

Flashlight Test

The size of the squint, which will determine the amount of surgery needed, can be measured by having the patient look at a flashlight while the examiner looks at the reflection of the light in the patient's eyes. The reflection will be off-center in the squinting eye. Each millimeter off-center equals 7° of 15 prism-diopters (degrees or prism-diopters are the standard units of squint measure [see Fig. 2-2]).

Cover Test

A second method of measuring squint is known as the cover test. While the patient looks at a target, cover the patient's straight eye with a card. The turned eye must then move to look at the test target. If the turned eye must turn in, the patient is an exotrope. The amount of compensatory movement gives the examiner an estimate of the size of the squint. To quantitate the compensatory movement, the examiner places prisms in front of the uncovered eye. The amount of prism that ultimately eliminates all compensatory movement equals the size of the squint. Thus, 35 prism-diopters of base-out prism means that the patient is afflicted with 35-prism-diopter esotropia.

Treating Esotropia

Corrective Lenses

Esotropic patients under 12 years of age who have amblyopia should be treated with a patch on the good eye until maximal improvement is observed in the amblyopic eye. The recommended treatment for accommodative esotropia is usually a full plus-spectacle correction. If the patient has a high accommodation:convergence ratio (i.e., if the esotropia is greater when the patient looks at a near target than when he looks at a far target), the strongest plus-spectacle correction tolerable to neutralize the accommodative effort at distance is prescribed along with eyedrops (e.g., Phospholine Iodide®) that contract the ciliary muscle so that accommodation (and thus convergence) is not necessary. Similarly, bifocal glasses lessen the need to accommodate for near vision and, thus, the need for excessive convergence.

Orthoptics

There are eye exercises designed to straighten a squint by strengthening the fusion processes in the brain. If fusion is not present, the exercises will not work. But in certain cases in which fusion is weakly present (e.g., intermittent exotropia or certain cases of partially accommodative esotropia), orthoptics revive and reeducate fusion.

Surgery

About 70% of all esotropes eventually require surgery, which is almost always performed under general anesthesia. The most common operation for esotropia is a weakening, or recession, of the medial rectus and a shortening, or resection, of the lateral rectus, both done in the esotropic eye. The amount of weakening required varies with the size of the squint. The results are not mathematically predictable, however, and the same surgery gives a larger effect in a larger angle of squint.

Surgical Prognosis. To evaluate the rate of surgical success, we must consider the prognosis of nonaccommodative esotropia without surgery and treatment. In a series of 122 children followed for 10 years without any treatment, the results were as follows:

15% became cosmetically acceptable

50% did not change

40% decreased the size of the squint somewhat

10% increased the size of the squint.[8]

The record of surgical success in the case of the typical nonaccommodating, nonfusing esotrope follows:

70% get good cosmetic results after one operation

80% get good cosmetic results after two operations.[9]

Alternating esotropia has a slightly poorer cosmetic prognosis.

Fusional results vary with many factors. Congenital esotropia has a very poor prognosis, but one school of thought maintains that if surgery is performed at age 6–18 months, many of the patients will achieve fusion.[10]

In a series of 26 intermittent esotropes with fusion, 50% achieved straight eyes and constant fusion without surgical correction.[11] In esotropia with onset between 3 and 5 years of age (when fusion has had a chance to develop), 70%–80% achieve fusion after surgery.[5] If we combine all types of esotropia, we find that about one-third achieve fusion after surgery. However, the overwhelming majority who attain fusion after treatment probably had developed it before the onset of squint.[12]

Diagnosing Exotropia

Twenty percent of all squint cases are exotropic. Of these, 85% are intermittent exotropes and thus have fusion. The condition first affects near vision, and gradually limits distance vision as well; it is generally not associated with any particular refractive error. The series of testing procedures is the same as that for esotropia.

Two facts should be kept in mind when evaluating the exotrope: (1) most are intermittent and thus use their fusion when their eyes are straight; and (2) most patients with exotropia have either the alternating or intermittent type, and so amblyopia is not a problem.

Treating Exotropia

In cases of intermittent exotropia, surgery is the treatment of choice if the squint becomes more constant as the child grows older. The surgery usually involves recessing the lateral rectus and resecting the medial rectus. If the exotropia is greater when the patient looks at a close object, however, recessions of the lateral recti of both eyes are performed. Thirty to fifty percent of exotropic patients achieve constant fusion after surgery,[13] and most achieve cosmetic success after surgery.[14]

Rationale

There are many legitimate approaches to the management of squint. The approach outlined in this chapter has been dictated by the cumulative demands of many parents of children with strabismus. And although we do not really know the causes of squint, we do know that, in cases other than accommodative squint, changing the position of the extraocular muscles surgically will more often than not make the child's eyes appear normal and allow the child to become socially accepted by his peers.

Does the surgical approach also bring fusion to the patient? We feel that fusion will be used by the child only if it was present at birth and if the eyes are straightened. Orthoptic exercises combined with surgery may often be of value; we feel, however, that there is a risk-benefit ratio, as there is with any treatment. If it appears that the cost of treatment and the risk of producing a psychologic cripple (a child overconcerned with his eyes) are too great, we do not advocate orthoptic exercises.

References

1. Waardenburg PJ, Franceschetti A, Klein D: *Genetics and Ophthalmology,* Vol II. The Netherlands, VanGorcum, N.V. Assen, 1963, p 1009

2. Frandsen AD: Occurrence of squint. Acta Ophthalmol [Suppl] (Kbh) 62:27, 1960

3. Moller PM: Influence of anesthesia and premedication on squint. Acta Ophthalmol (Kbh) 36:499, 1958

4. Duke-Elder S: *System of Ophthalmology,* Vol VI. *Ocular Motility and Strabismus.* St. Louis, Mosby, 1973, pp 223–228

5. Lyle TK: Treatment of concomitant convergent strabismus. Trans Ophthalmol Soc UK 72:403, 1952

6. Houlton ACL: Treatment of concomitant convergent strabismus. Trans Ophthalmol Soc UK 72:397, 1952

7. Francois J, James J: Comparative study of amblyopic treatment. Am Orthopt J, 5:61, 1955

8. Nordlow W: Spontaneous changes in refraction and angle of squint together with the state of retinal correspondence and visual acuity in concomitant convergent strabismus during years of growth. Acta Ophthalmol (Kbh) 29:383, 1951

9. Dunnington JH, Regan EF: Factors influencing the postoperative results in concomitant convergent strabismus. Arch Ophthalmol 44:813, 1950

10. Costenbader FD: Infantile esotropia. Trans Am Ophthalmol Soc 59:397, 1961

11. Duke-Elder: p 472

12. Sashell GTW: Long-term results of treatment of concomitant convergent strabismus in terms of binocular function. Trans Ophthalmol Soc UK 72:367, 1952

13. Lyle TK, Foley J: Prognosis in cases of strabismus with special reference to orthoptic treatment. Br J Ophthalmol 41:129, 1957

14. Dunlap EA, Gaffney RD: Surgical management of intermittent exotropia. Am Orthopt J 13:20, 1963

Chapter 11

Retinal Disease

It can be said that the retina represents the ultimate level of sophistication in the evolution of biologic tissue. It can both detect a few quanta of light and process a complex visual scene, transmitting the biologic equivalent of up to half a billion bits (a computer unit) of information per second over the optic nerve.[1] Such complexity parallels that of the brain. Indeed, the retina is an outgrowth of the embryonic forebrain; its layering of nerve cells and nerve fibers follows the brain's pattern of white nerve-fibers and gray nerve-cell bodies (Fig. 1-11).

Nature's price for such complexity is rapid energy turnover. The retina uses oxygen and glucose at a rate higher than any other tissue in the body.[2] Since these substances are supplied by both the retinal and choroidal circulations, the amount of blood-flow per unit time, per gram of tissue, in this area is also the greatest in the body.[3]

Given its high metabolic rate, the retina is vulnerable to disease. Its healthy function depends primarily on the integrity of its blood supply and on a full complement of all the enzymes needed to keep the visual processes operating at this rapid rate. It is not surprising, then, that the most common retinal disease is *diabetic retinopathy,* a condition in which many of the retinal capillaries occlude or rupture. In either instance, sections of the retina die as a result of inadequate blood supply. In *hypertensive retinopathy,* many of the small arterioles of the retina constrict, again resulting in retinal infarcts.

Within the retina itself, the macula demonstrates an even more exaggerated response to systemic and local vascular disease.[4] Although the reason for this exaggerated response is not known, the area does have some anatomic peculiarities. First, the vascular arcade, hovering over the avascular *foveola* (the center of the fovea), may act as a watershed in which wastes collect faster than in surrounding tissue. Second, while Müller fibers normally run in a columnar fashion from vitreous surface to pigment epithelium, supporting the retina, these fibers run horizontally in the macula, allowing tissue laxity and easier accumulation of fluid. Finally, the yellow pigment of the macula tends to absorb large amounts of energy in the ultraviolet and blue portions of the light spectrum. In cases of aphakia, the normal filter for the blue end of the spectrum is lost, and high concentrations of this short-wavelength energy may induce damage in genetically susceptible individuals.

Before discussing retinal disease, however, we must gain an appreciation of one of our most important diagnostic tools.

Fluorescein Angiography

As our ophthalmoscopes improve, with better optics and brighter illumination, we are allowed to see the more subtle pathologic changes of the fundus. Conventional ophthalmoscopy, however, cannot show us the dynamics of pathology—only its results. Specifically, the normal retinal vasculature, as part of the blood-brain barrier, does not leak. In such conditions as diabetes, serum may leak from microaneurysms, but the leakage of clear serum is invisible to the ophthalmoscope. Only significant leakage leading to sizeable edema results in retinal change that can be seen through the ophthalmoscope. Again, it is normal for serum to leak continually from the choriocapillaris, but the tight junctions between retinal pigment epithelium prevent seepage into the retina. If the pigment epithelium is diseased, seepage into the retina occurs, but cannot be seen with the ophthalmoscope until sizeable edema or actual retinal detachment has occurred.

One of the truly great advances in diagnostic ophthalmology was the development of fluorescein angiography. In the late 1950s, Milton Flocks at Stanford injected fluorescein into the veins of normal cats and recorded, photographically, the passage of the fluoresceinated blood as it flowed within the transparent walls of the arteries and veins.[5] In 1960, Edward Maumanee, the director of the Wilmer Institute at Johns Hopkins University, placed a blue filter over his ophthalmoscope and injected fluorescein into the vein of a human patient with a tumor of the choroid. Dr. Maumanee vividly described how the dye filled the abnormal blood spaces of the choroidal hemangioma.[6] Finally, in 1960 two medical students, H. Novotny and D. Alvis, while on a three-month elective in medical physiology, experimented first on themselves and then on patients with diabetes; they worked out a reproducible technique for taking high-quality, high-speed fluorescein angiophotographs of the retina. Their original photographs clearly demonstrated the abnormal leakage from the retinal circulation of the diabetic patient.[7] It was a fortuitous combination of profoundly professional researchers, enthusiastic amateurs, and sage clinicians that gave fluorescein angiography to the clinical community.

Diabetic Retinopathy

In 1974, more than 600,000 new cases of diabetes were diagnosed, and the incidence of diabetes appears to be increasing by 6% per year.[8] At this rate, the number of people with diabetes will double in 15 years. This means that the average American born today has a better-than-one-in-five chance of developing the disease. Concomitantly, in 1974 diabetic retinopathy became the leading cause of blindness in this country.

A patient usually has diabetes for 10 to 20 years before the retina is affected. At present 38% of the diabetic population has some degree of retinopathy. Diabetic retinopathy was not a major problem before the development of insulin therapy by Banting and Best in 1921, because most diabetics died soon after the onset of their disease. As treatment improves, the diabetic patient lives longer. That is, his heart, brain, and kidneys survive longer, but the retina frequently becomes progressively compromised. Insulin, proper diet, and oral hypoglycemic agents all seem to slow the pace of the systemic disease. As renal circulation is slowly compromised, a functional accommodation takes place (after all, most humans can function normally with the equivalent of only one kidney). But the retina is too compact and too tiny and its organization too high-powered to tolerate even minor insults.

Pathology

Pathologic changes occur primarily in the retina, rather than in the choroidal capillaries, and thus the disease affects the inner half of the retina. Thickening of the capillary basement-membrane with closure of capillaries is an important finding. The loss of capillary pericytes (which normally encase the capillary in a supporting mesh) is another fundamental pathologic change, and the loss of pericytes leads to a weakening in the structural integrity of the capillary wall, producing microaneurysms. Closure of capillaries can produce swelling and death in the retinal nerve fibers supplied by those capillaries. The resulting lesions are called *cotton-wool infarcts* because they appear swollen and gray-white when viewed with the ophthalmoscope. Intraretinal leakage from these damaged capillaries can present as exudate or edema, or, if the porosity of the capillary increases sufficiently, as hemorrhage. If regions of capillary closure are widespread, the adjacent oxygen-deprived retinal tissue probably elaborates a vasoproliferative factor.[911] New vessels begin to grow over the surface of the retina and disc and onto the postvitreous face.

There are two categories of diabetic retinopathy. *Nonproliferative diabetic retinopathy* develops insidiously, gradually decreasing visual acuity, and occurs most often in association with adult-onset diabetes. Visual acuity rarely deteriorates beyond 20/400. *Proliferative diabetic retinopathy* is seen more commonly in juvenile diabetes and can lead to total blindness both from intractable vitreous hemorrhage or fibrosis of the neovascular tissue and from the production of recalcitrant retinal detachment. Table 11-1 outlines the progression of diabetic retinopathy.

Treatment

In the mid-1960s, Drs. William Beetham and Lloyd Aiello, of the Joslin Clinic in Boston, noted that those diabetics who had extensive scarring and retinal atrophy from old chorioretinitis, as well as those with extensive myopic degeneration of the retina or retinitis pigmentosa, did not develop severe diabetic retinopathy. Beetham and Aiello reasoned that since diabetes was a disease of small blood vessels, large areas of atrophy meant that less retinal tissue had to be nourished by the faltering blood supply. Why not destroy large, unimportant areas of the severe diabetic's retina with a laser? The spot size of the early ruby laser beam was small enough that the surgeon could destroy one-half of the retina (avoiding the macular area), while hardly disturbing the nerve-fiber layer and inducing no major visual-field defects. There was a significant improvement in vision despite the diabetic retinopathy.[12] Since then, the argon laser has proven to be even more helpful in treatment (Fig. 11-1).[13]

Laser or other forms of photocoagulation produce localized retinal destruction, with a resultant decrease in retinal oxygen requirements. Theoretically, both the total amount of oxygen-dependent retina and the need for new vessels is then reduced. We have no proof for the theory, but the fact remains that such treatment is followed in most cases by regression of the neovascularization. In some severe cases, however, the disease process is unyielding and fibrovascular proliferation continues, producing severe hemorrhage and retinal detachments.

Patients with proliferative diabetic retinopathy are beset with other problems as well. They often suffer severe kidney disease. Some will develop new blood vessels in the filtering angle of the eye, resulting in unremitting neovascular glaucoma. Finally, the appearance of proliferative retinopathy signals a significantly shorter life expectancy. For example, 25% of patients with proliferative diabetic retinopathy are dead within two years of the diagnosis, 50% are dead within five years, and 75% are dead within 10 years.

A summary of suggested ophthalmic care for diabetic retinopathy follows:

1. Internist should dilate pupil and examine fundus yearly.

Table 11-1. Progressive Stages of Diabetic Retinopathy and Associated Clinical Findings[a]

Stage	Clinical Findings
No evidence of retinopathy (10+ years)	None
Background retinopathy	Few scattered round hemorrhages (RHs) or microaneurysms
	Few hard exudates
	Minimal venous changes
Accelerated retinopathy	Drop in ERG oscillatory potentials
	Cotton-wool spots
	Many RHs and microaneurysms
	Retinal edema
	Moderate to marked venous changes (tortuosity and segmental changes such as bleeding)
Proliferative retinopathy	New vessels (neovascularization)
	Preretinal and vitreal hemorrhages
Retinitis proliferans	Gliosis/fibrosis appears
	Hemorrhages continue
	Secondary problems such as: Macular traction Retinal detachment Rubeosis iridis (glaucoma)
Quiescent phase	Hemorrhages diminish
	Destructive process ends
	Secondary problems may continue

[a]Courtesy of Dr. J. Weiter.

2. If vision drops or evidence of retinopathy is present, the patient should be referred to an ophthalmologist.

3. Yearly photos of fundus should be taken.

4. Any patient with neovascularization or macular edema should undergo fluorescein angiography.

5. When maculopathy or neovascularization occurs in specific areas, the physician should seriously consider argon-laser photocoagulation.

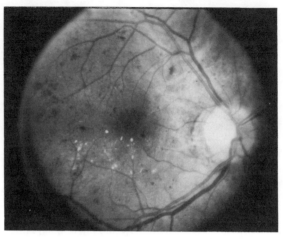

Figure 11-1. Photograph of the retina in a case of nonproliferative diabetic retinopathy. *White areas:* fatty, hard exudates. *Dark areas:* hemorrhages. (Courtesy of Dr. J. Weiter.)

A Case of Nonproliferative Diabetic Retinopathy

A 54-year-old lawyer noticed a gradual difficulty in reading his briefs and contracts. His optometrist could not improve the poor visual acuity with glasses and referred the patient for ophthalmologic evaluation. The man had been afflicted with diabetes for ten years and was diet-controlled.

Visual acuity was:

RE 20/100
LE 20/80

The patient had minimal lens opacification. Retinal examination through dilated pupils revealed typical background diabetic retinopathy (Fig. 11-1) with hard shiny exudates, dot hemorrhages (blood in deep retinal layers), flame hemorrhages (blood trapped in nerve-fiber layer), red dots (microaneurysms), and general pallor (diffuse retinal edema) throughout the macular region.

Fluorescein angiography (Fig. 11-2) showed diffuse leakage of fluorescein (representing serum) from abnormally permeable capillaries and microaneurysms. This serum leakage leads to retinal edema, separating and distorting the retinal elements and decreasing visual acuity.

Treatment. Local laser destruction of the leakage sites can decrease the amount of edema formation and improve the visual acuity in some cases. In most cases, the treatment is simply watchful waiting, for some cases will improve spontaneously.

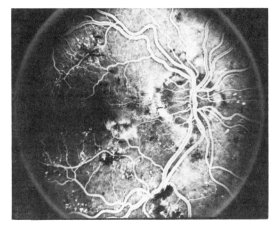

Figure 11-2. Fluorescein angiogram of the patient in Figure 11-1. All blood vessels are outlined by the fluorescein dye, which leaks from the microaneurysms. (Courtesy of Dr. J. Weiter.)

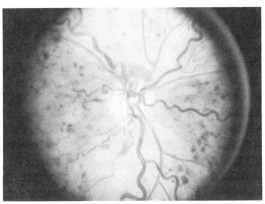

Figure 11-3. Photograph of the retina of a patient with proliferative diabetic retinopathy, as seen with the ophthalmoscope. Twisting new vessels are seen on the surface of the optic nerve along with the proliferating fibrous tissue. (Courtesy of Dr. J. Weiter.)

A Case of Proliferative Diabetic Retinopathy

A 26-year-old ski instructor was involved in a slalom competition when she noticed the spontaneous onset of a black floater in the periphery of the visual field of her right eye. This disappeared slowly over the next few days. She had been an insulin-dependent juvenile diabetic for the past 13 years. A routine medical and eye examination that week had indicated that she was in excellent condition. Two weeks later, however, she awakened to notice a total blur in the right eye. When the blur failed to clear, she immediately consulted her ophthalmologist. Visual acuity was:

RE counting fingers at 2 feet
LE 20/20

On retinal examination through the dilated pupil of her right eye, the retina could not be visualized because of a dense vitreous hemorrhage. The retina of the left eye showed severe neovascular proliferation from the optic nerve head (Fig. 11-3), and fluorescein angiography of the left eye revealed leakage along all of the new vessels (Fig. 11-4). One can surmise from this left eye that a similar condition existed in the right eye and that the new vessels had bled into the vitreous cavity. The small floater that occurred two weeks before was probably a small hemorrhage from the new blood vessels which spontaneously resorbed. The latter vitreous hemorrhage was a catastrophic bleed.

This case represents the most severe type of diabetic retinopathy (proliferative). There is new vessel formation secondary to hypoxia (the result of capillary shutdown). The new vessels cannot grow through the tightly knit retinal tissue, but instead climb onto the face of the retina from around the edge of the optic nerve onto the surface of the vitreous. With movement of the head or slight trauma, the vitreous tends to shear these new vessels, producing the resultant bleeding.

Treatment. Pan-retinal laser photocoagulation as described by Beetham and Aiello (Fig. 11-5). [12,13]

Retinal Trauma

When a fist or a ball strikes the eye, the shock-wave that develops in the ocular fluid can injure the retina in three ways. The wave, transmitted through the vitreous, slaps the retina. Such a blow induces retinal swelling *(contra-coup injury)*. Second, as the wave reflects off the back of the eye, the vitreous pulls on the retina wherever it is anatomically attached. If there is a firm attachment to the wall of a blood vessel, for example, the vessel may be torn open after the vitreal wave ricochets off the back of the eye. Finally, since the vitreous is normally attached to areas of the retina, the reflected wave may tear the retina itself.

A Case of Traumatic Vitreous Hemorrhage

An 18-year-old boy was playing in a collegiate championship tennis match when his opponent's serve bounced up and struck him solidly in the left eye. He noted immediate blurring of visual acuity and was promptly taken

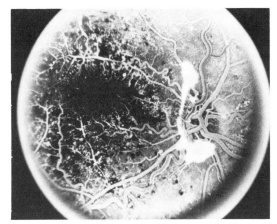

Figure 11-4. Fluorescein angiogram of patient in Figure 11-3. Note the leakage of fluorescein from all of the new blood vessels. (Courtesy of Dr. J. Weiter.)

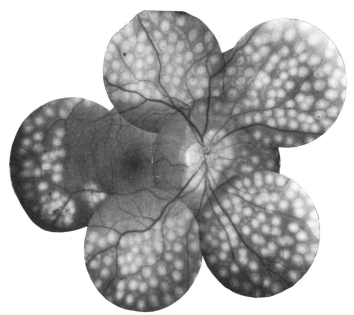

Figure 11-5. Composite photograph of a patient with diabetic retinopathy 24 hours after panretinal photocoagulation. (Courtesy of Retina Associates of Boston.)

to the office of an ophthalmologist. He had no previous history or family history of retinal disease.

Visual acuity was:

RE 20/20
LE light perception

A slit-lamp examination showed the anterior aspect of the eyes to be normal. The posterior aspect of the right eye, as examined with the ophthalmoscope, was normal. When the left eye was examined, however, the view of the retina was obscured by dense retinal hemorrhage.

Treatment. He was sent home with both eyes bandaged, placed on strict bed rest, and told to sleep on three pillows. The rationale of such therapy is that when both eyes are patched, the patient is less interested in his environment and tends to move around less. With the head elevated, gravity helps settle the blood to the bottom of the eye and out of the visual axis.

Two weeks after the injury, the vitreous hemorrhage had already cleared by about 75% and the visual acuity was 20/30. The retina could be seen easily (Figs. 11-6 and 11-7). Examination of his peripheral retina revealed a superior nasal retinal detachment, which was the result of the retina pulling away from its usual mooring at the ora serrata. (A tear is called a *dialysis* if it occurs at the natural seam along the ora serrata.) This was treated successfully with surgery. Six months postoperatively, his visual acuity was 20/20, the retina was attached, and the vitreous was clear.

The cause of the vitreous hemorrhage was secondary disruption of a retinal vessel by force. This usually clots spontaneously in a short period of time. Only when the vitreous clears is the ophthalmologist able to identify the source of the bleed.

This case underscores the point that with concussion or contusion injuries it is very important to examine periodically the peripheral retina for up to one year after the injury. In most cases the vitreous blood clears without further problems. In some cases, however, the injury pulls on the vitreous, which in turn pulls off the retina at the ora serrata and causes a retinal dialysis. The retina will detach, however, only when the fluid vitreous slowly leaks under the retina and balloons it forward, and this may take months to develop.

In other cases there may be abnormal vitreo-retinal adhesions present in other parts of the retina prior to trauma. Vitreous traction in the region of the adhesion produces a retinal tear, and detachment occurs when the liquid vitreous seeps through that tear.

A Case of Traumatic Retinal Edema

A 52-year-old art thief was struck over the head and face while involved in a robbery attempt. Dazed and blurry-eyed, he was apprehended by the police. When he reported diminished vision in the right eye, the prison guards arranged an appointment with an ophthalmologist.

Visual acuity was:

RE 20/200
LE 20/20

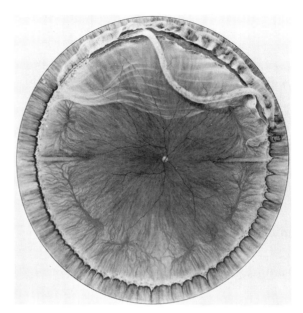

Figure 11-6. Drawing of the peripheral retina as seen with the indirect ophthalmoscope. Note the area of the retina pulled from its insertion at the ora serrata. This is known as a *retinal dialysis*. These cases often proceed to retinal detachment. (Reprinted with permission from Weidenthal D, Schepens CL: Peripheral fundus change associated with contusion. Am J Ophthalmol 62:465, 1966.)

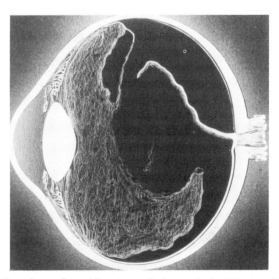

Figure 11-7. Drawing of a side view of the retinal dialysis of Figure 11-6. (Courtesy of Retina Associates of Boston. Artist: David Tilden.)

Ophthalmoscopic examination of the right eye showed the vitreous to be clear, but the retina in the macula region looked grayish, with loss of the normal foveal reflection, and a few small extrafoveal hemorrhages were noted. The left eye was normal. The primary pathologic alteration in this area is one of *intraretinal edema* secondary to the shock, or contra-coup, injury.

Treatment. There is no treatment for this condition other than time. The visual acuity usually returns to normal, as it did in this case, but occasionally some macular scarring results in permanent loss of sharp vision.

Retinitis Pigmentosa

This tragic disease affects less than 0.5% of the population.[14] For reasons still not well understood, the rods and cones do not function normally, and with each passing year an increasing number of these photoreceptors die. As the disease progresses, the patient's visual world narrows, until all peripheral vision is gone. Ultimately, central vision disappears as well.

A Case of Retinitis Pigmentosa

A 25-year-old stewardess had noted difficulty seeing at dusk since she was a teenager. The condition had become "maddening" while driving at dusk and worse at night. She denied any predisposing or precipitating factor, and her family history was negative.

Visual acuity was:

RE 20/20
LE 20/20

The anterior aspects of both eyes were normal, but the ophthalmoscope revealed a slight thinning of the retinal vessels. Collections of black pigment-clumps had formed a bone-spicule pattern in the middle retina, and the head of the optic nerve looked pale (Fig. 11-8). A visual-field examination showed a blind area in the form of a large ring about 20 degrees off center (Fig. 11-9), and an electroretinogram (ERG), which measures the electrical activity of the eye, revealed diminished activity of the rods and cones.

Treatment. There is presently no treatment for retinitis pigmentosa.

Discussion. Since the disease initially attacks the retinal midperiphery (the area of macula and optic nerve are not affected until later in the disease), the rods, which are the most common element in that region, are

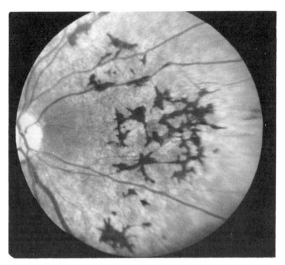

Figure 11-8. Picture of the posterior pole of the retina in a patient with retinitis pigmentosa, as seen with the ophthalmoscope. Note the "bone spicule" pattern of the collections of black pigment, the attenuated blood vessels, and the appearance of the optic nerve. (Courtesy of Dr. E. Berson.)

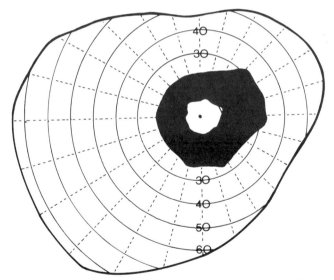

Figure 11-9. Example of the typical midperipheral ring scotoma (blind area) seen in a patient with retinitis pigmentosa. (Artist: Laurel Cook.)

affected first. Because the rods are responsible for night vision, patients such as the one just described report difficulty seeing in the dark. As the disease progresses and more of the retina dies, side vision is lost and the patient often bumps into walls and furniture. As the rods and cones succumb, they are replaced by black scar tissue that accumulates along atrophied branching blood vessels (accounting for the black bone-spicule formations seen with the ophthalmoscope).

Retinal Detachment

The ever-hungry retinal energy machine is fueled by the retinal circulation that supplies the inner layers closest to the vitreous and by the choroidal circulation that feeds the pigment epithelium and the photoreceptors in the outer half of the retina. If part of the retina is lifted away from the choroidal circulation, that part of the retina loses its ability to record detailed imagery. In fact, a tear in the retina can develop, and fluid, primarily from the vitreous, can seep between the pigment epithelium and the rod and cone layer, and balloon the retina into the vitreous cavity away from the choroidal circulation. Traumatic detachment has been described. Retinal tears, with subsequent detachment, can result from severe myopia as well. The elongated shape of the eye in some severe myopes results in elevated tension between the vitreous and the retina, and in some cases the attachments give way and vitreous flows behind the retina.

Treatment

The history of retinal detachment is filled with mysticism and incorrect theories. In 1841, before the ophthalmoscope was invented, Sichel recognized it as a gray membrane with blood vessels behind the pupil.[15] Nevertheless, retinal detachment was not understood until the ophthalmoscope was invented and then accepted as a legitimate tool of diagnosis.

In 1870, Wecker and Jaeger concluded that a retinal break was essential in causing a retinal detachment.[16] But what produced the breaks? In 1882, Leber suggested that changes in the vitreous too fine to be seen caused these breaks.[17] As one can imagine, a hypothesis suggesting that invisible changes in the vitreous produced the condition were severely ridiculed, and Leber ultimately changed his mind.[18] But in 1920 the Swiss ophthalmologist Jules Gonin clearly demonstrated the relationship between the vitreous body and a retinal tear and developed a treatment for detached retina.[19] He cauterized the area of the sclera in the region of the hole in an attempt to produce a scar around the tear. After a series of successful retinal reattachments, he presented his material to the world. He reasoned that if one could fix this region of the tear in place by scarification, the subretinal fluid would resorb and the retina would become reattached. If a tear (rupture) is not closed or scarred, then the detachment tends to perpetuate and extend.

Tears in the peripheral retina can be of varying sizes and types, and are usually associated with retinal degeneration. The tears do not occur in the healthy eye, except in cases of trauma. They are usually associated with such degenerative processes in the vitreous and retina as old inflammation, senility, or myopic degeneration. They may also follow cataract extraction, in which case the vitreous comes forward, occupying the space of the extracted lens. The forward movement of the vitreous may pull on the retina, producing a tear. With age, the vitreous gradually changes from a gel to a liquid state. If there are any vitreo-retinal adhesions (such adhesions are not normal) present when the solid vitreous collapses, it pulls on the retina, producing a tear. Liquid vitreous then seeps through the tear separating the retina from the pigment epithelium. Ten percent of those patients with retinal detachment in one eye will ultimately develop the condition in the other eye.[20]

Surgical Procedures

After identifying the tears, as Gonin noted, the treatment of a retinal detachment basically consists of producing a scar surrounding the tears (by welding the retina to the pigment epithelium with thermal injury) so that liquid vitreous can no longer leak beneath the retina. This task is not as easy as it may sound. Before operating one must make an exhaustive search to identify and locate all retinal holes. This is done with indirect ophthalmoscopy and scleral depression. Scleral depression is performed by indenting the sclera so that the peripheral retina can be seen and evaluated (Fig. 11-10).

In most cases the surgeon can easily surround the tears with inflammation produced by an extremely cold probe *(cryotherapy)* or a very hot probe *(diathermy)* passed through the sclera. Often, the surgeon must add a step to the procedure. If the vitreous traction that initiated the original tear is great, the area of the tear must be indented forward for two reasons: to slacken the traction and to reunite the retina to the pigment epithelium so that the scarring around the tear can take place. This can be accomplished with the aid of a small silicone-sponge implant pleated on the sclera over the tear or, if the situation necessitates it, an encircling band tightened around the entire globe to indent the implant even farther (Fig. 11-11). If the tear is still not approximating the retinal pigment epithelium because of the subretinal fluid, the fluid must be cautiously drained. The success rate of modern retinal reattachment surgery is approximately 85%.[21] Fortunately, retinal detachment is rare, occurring in only one out of 10,000 people.[22,23] Retinal detachment is about 20 times more common in the white population than in the black population.[24]

A Case of Retinal Detachment

A 55-year-old, severely myopic professor of physics was looking out the window one evening when he noted some flashes of lightning. Oddly enough, no one else in his family noticed them. As the week progressed,

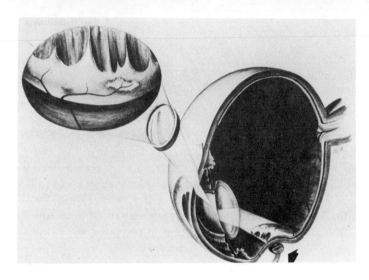

Figure 11-10. Method of examining the peripheral retina using scleral depression and the binocular indirect ophthalmoscope. The scleral depressor *(arrow)* indents the eye so that the retinal periphery is brought into view. The insert shows the appearance of the ora serrata. (Courtesy of Retina Associates of Boston. Artist: W. Stenstrom.)

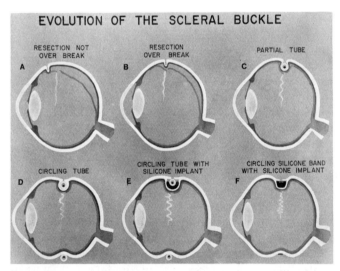

Figure 11-11. Various steps in the development of the scleral buckling technique. First the original lamellar scleral resection **(A)** was modified so that it was performed over the retinal break **(B)**. Later, a partial polyethylene tube was inserted under the resection sutures to create a buckle effect **(C)**. This was followed by the introduction of an encircling polyethylene tube for buckle permanency **(D)**. Silicone implants were later added under the tubing to create a wider buckle **(E)**. Finally, the tubing was replaced by a soft elastic silicone rubber band **(F)**. (Reprinted with permission from Schepens CL, Regan C (eds): *Controversial Aspects of the Management of Retinal Detachment.* Boston, Little Brown, 1965, p 116.)

so did the occurrence of these flashes, which seemed to take the shape of an arc of a circle. Then he noticed little specks floating across his line of sight. The following week, as he faced his class, a curtain appeared to descend between him and all of the students in the right balcony. He quickly consulted his ophthalmologist.

His visual acuity was:

RE counting fingers
LE 20/20

The anterior aspect of both eyes was normal. An ophthalmoscopic examination revealed a gray-white elevated detachment of the left lower retina of the right eye. After the pupils were dilated, the peripheral retina revealed a tear. The left fundus showed some narrowing and straightening out of the retinal vessels and a large crescent of retinal atrophy adjacent to the optic nerve—findings typical of high myopia.

Treatment. The patient underwent surgery, and three months postoperatively recorded a visual acuity of 20/25 in the right eye.

Discussion. This history is typical of a patient who develops a retinal tear from traction by the vitreous at the peripheral vitreo-retinal adhesion. The perception of lightning flashes are secondary to the retina being pulled on by the vitreous adhesion, and the floaters are caused by a small amount of bleeding from ruptured retinal vessels. The curtain phenomenon is secondary to gradual leakage of liquid vitreous beneath the retina, and gravity augments the separation of the retina.

Flashes and Floaters—Vitreous Detachment

One of the more common complaints of patients who seek ophthalmologic help is that of seeing "dark, floating specks and lines" or of seeing flashes of light. In 85% of cases, the problem is located in the vitreous.[25] Most of the time, the onset of symptoms signals a splitting of the posterior vitreous face (internal limiting membrane) into two layers. A defect in the inner layer allows the rapid passage of liquefied vitreous into the newly formed retrovitreous space. As a result, the two layers become separated; the outer layer remains attached to the retina, but the inner layer becomes detached. The main mass of solid vitreous then collapses and sinks inferiorly. This is known as a *posterior vitreous detachment.* After a posterior vitreous detachment, vitreous traction on the retina may produce the sensation of a light flash, or a tear in a retinal capillary may produce a tiny or sizeable hemorrhage that might cause the sensation of a dark, floating speck or line. The sensation of seeing floating lines or specks may also be caused by strands of solid vitreous floating in a local pool of liquid vitreous, again as the result of the disruption of the homogeneity of the vitreous caused by its collapse. Finally, vitreous traction can produce retinal tears.

Since combined symptoms of seeing flashes and floaters can be associated with serious retinal disease, such patients should be referred for a thorough retinal examination by an ophthalmologist. If no treatable disease is found, the patient is assured that the floaters will probably sink out of sight, but yearly reevaluation of the retina is important in discovering new problems as they arise. It should be noted that the complaint of an occasional floater, seen in one or both eyes, does not necessitate an ophthalmic evaluation unless the patient displays a significant amount of apprehension.

Senile Macular Degeneration

The macula is the part of the retina adapted to seeing details most clearly. Vision in this area is responsible for our ability to identify faces, to read fine print, and to discern various shades of color. Macular (central) vision functions best in the daylight.

The macula is more vulnerable to disease and degeneration than any other part of the retina. For example, 30% of adults over the age of 65 have some degree of macular degeneration, and it is considered to be the most common cause of legal blindness in the elderly in England.[26]

This area of the retina is more vulnerable to degeneration than the rest of the retina because of the requirements of the pigment epithelium. The single-cell layer of pigment epithelium appears to be the key to the health of the retinal elements in the macula, regulating the transfer of nutrients to the photoreceptors and removing waste products. In this region the pigment epithelium is taller and appears to contain more pigment than other regions, as observed during fluorescein angiography. It seems to have a greater need for oxygen and other nutrients than other parts of the retina. We suggest that its higher degree of pigmentation absorbs more light, and requires a more efficient cooling system, than other retinal areas.[26,27] These needs are fulfilled by the vessels of the adjacent choroid. Indeed, pathologic specimens taken at autopsy from patients who had senile macular degeneration reveal thickening of the choroidal-vessel walls. This thickening can interfere with cooling, slow down the supply of vital elements to the macular region, and lead to a slow degeneration of the overlying pigment epithelium. Senile macular degeneration involves both eyes, but usually develops at different rates in the two; the progress is usually gradual, but there may be periods of accelerated deterioration.

A Case of Senile Macular Degeneration

A 67-year-old draftsman noticed that it was increasingly difficult for him to distinguish the divisions of his micrometer. His general health was good, but the vision in his left eye had been poor for approximately 10 years. Although his family doctor advised him to have it checked by an ophthalmologist, he could never find the time. Now that the visual acuity of his right eye was also decreasing, with an associated distortion of street signs, he sought the help of an ophthalmologist.

The examination revealed the following:

Visual acuity	RE 20/30
	LE hand movement
Anterior aspect both eyes	Normal
Ophthalmoscope: RE	Multiple drusen in the macular area with a shallow detachment of the retina centrally
Ophthalmoscope: LE	Dense central subretinal fibrotic scar with surrounding hemorrhage (Figs. 11-12, 11-13)

The patient's left eye had lost all of its central vision because of the bleeding beneath the retina and because of the subsequent formation of scars. His right eye had a localized subretinal leakage of fluid through the abnormal retinal pigment epithelium.

Treatment. Such a patient must be examined as soon as possible with fluorescein angiography. If the areas of leakage are not in the central macula, the condition may be amenable to focal laser photocoagulation, which will destroy the region of abnormal permeability. This may prevent further leakage and allow the macula to assume its normal position.

Discussion. With aging there is sclerosis of the choriocapillaris and thickening of the basement (Bruch's) membrane of the pigment epithelium. Nodular excrescences build up on the inner portion of this membrane. The etiology is still obscure, but the excrescences are thought to be metabolic debris from the overlying retinal pigment epithelium. They are clearly visible with the ophthalmoscope as grayish-yellow lesions and are called *drusen* (from the Greek, meaning nodule). The drusen alone usually produce no decrease in visual acuity. Only when the retinal pigment epithelium begins to degenerate over the drusen do the visual problems appear. As the intercellular bridges of the retinal pigment epithelium break down, fluid from the choriocapillaris can pass readily

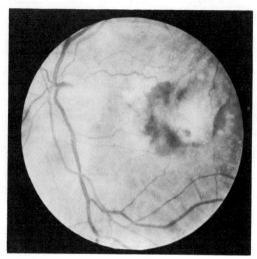

Figure 11-12. Photograph of retina with senile, hemorrhagic, macular degeneration. Note the central scar surrounded by hemorrhage. (Courtesy of Dr. J. Weiter.)

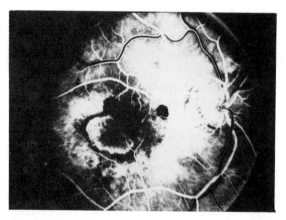

Figure 11-13. Fluorescein angiogram of patient in Figure 11-12. (Courtesy of Dr. J. Weiter.)

beneath the retina. When the macular retina becomes separated from the retinal pigment epithelium, visual acuity is decreased.

If the situation is present for some time, the body appears to make an abortive effort to get blood to the separated macula. Specifically, new vessels from the choriocapillaris can form, breaking through Bruch's membrane and developing a network just beneath the retina.[27] Unfortunately, the new vessels leak serum or bleed, detaching the macula even more. If chronic serum leakage or bleeding occurs in the central macula, the condition will eventually produce a scar and total loss of central visual acuity. The condition is usually unremitting. The disease does not always follow this sequence. Often the process is so slow that all one can see is a slow death of pigment epithelium and a consequent decrease in visual acuity.

Tumors

Tumors of the retina (retinoblastoma) and underlying choroid (choroidal melanomas) are relatively rare in ophthalmology.

Retinoblastoma is a tumor of childhood and presents as *leukocoria* (white pupil). The diagnosis is made by the age of three in approximately 85% of cases.[28] Thirty-five percent of the cases are bilateral. Early diagnosis and treatment will prevent extraocular extension and eventual death. The prognosis is excellent if the condition is uniocular and localized in the eye tissue.

Choroidal melanoma, on the other hand, is by far the most common intraocular tumor, with an overall incidence of from 5 to 7.5 cases per million a year.[29] It is nonhereditary, rarely bilateral, and almost never seen in black patients. The tumor is derived from melanocytes in the choroidal stroma. It may occur near the macula and affect visual acuity, or it may arise peripherally and enlarge to a great size before it becomes symptomatic.

A Case of Retinoblastoma

A 7-month-old girl was taken to an ophthalmologist with a white pupil in her left eye, which, according to her mother, had been present for a month. The child was examined under light anesthesia after both pupils were maximally dilated, and the examination revealed white lesions splashed over the retina (Fig. 11-14). This clinical picture was consistent with the diagnosis of retinoblastoma.

Treatment. Typically, in such cases, treatment consists of enucleation if the tumor is in only one eye. If the condition is bilateral, the more involved eye is enucleated and the other eye undergoes radiotherapy. If the condition recurs, the ophthalmologist photocoagulates the tumors. Those patients who survive the hereditary variety of retinoblastoma may be at higher risk (10% or greater) of developing subsequent childhood cancer.[30]

A Case of Choroidal Melanoma

A 62-year-old Iranian prince was referred to an American ophthalmologist for treatment of distorted vision in his left eye, a condition that had

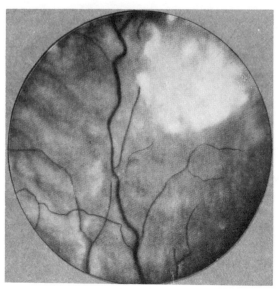

Figure 11-14. Photograph of the retina of a patient with retinoblastoma. (Courtesy of Dr. E. Ryan.)

been present for a year. His medical history was somewhat confused, but through his large retinue of interpreters and servants the ophthalmologist was able to learn that the prince was otherwise in good health.

Visual acuity was:

RE 20/20
LE 20/30 (with marked distortion)

Indirect ophthalmoscopy demonstrated that the right eye was normal, but the left eye had a large and slightly elevated gray lesion just superior to and involving the central fovea (Fig. 11-15). Fluorescein angiography revealed diffuse leakage from the lesion about 40 minutes after the dye was injected. The diagnosis—malignant melanoma of the choroid—was confirmed by a radioactive P_{32} uptake examination.

Diagnostic Approach. When a suspicious lesion is seen in the fundus, the following questions should be raised and answered:

1. Is the lesion a malignant choroidal melanoma?

2. If the lesion is malignant, what is the proper treatment?

3. If the eye is enucleated and examined microscopically, what are the probabilities for patient survival?

The diagnosis of malignant melanoma of the choroid can be made with a high degree of accuracy by using only clinical tests. Differential

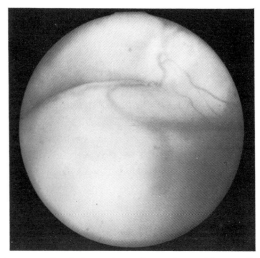

Figure 11-15. Photograph of the retina of a patient with a malignant melanoma. Note the smooth elevated edge of the lesion. (Courtesy of Retina Associates of Boston.)

diagnosis includes subretinal hemorrhage, benign nevus, choroidal detachment, benign angioma, and various pigmented degenerations. Naturally, the expertise of the examiner will influence the diagnostic accuracy. The rate of successful diagnosis, averaged from the world literature, is 95%.[28]

The following steps lead to the clinical diagnosis:

1. The lesion is first observed through a dilated pupil with the indirect ophthalmoscope. This test alone successfully diagnoses the lesion in over 85% of the cases.[31]

2. Transillumination of the globe while observing the dilated pupil will often confirm an ophthalmoscopic impression, since solid pigmented tumors and subretinal hemorrhages do not transilluminate.

3. To confirm the ophthalmoscopic impression, ophthalmic ultrasonography is usually the next step. A solid tumor of greater than 2 mm elevation produces a characteristically low internal reflectivity profile, which is correctly diagnosed more than 85% of the time by an experienced ultrasonographer.[32]

4. If the diagnosis is still equivocal, a fluorescein angiogram should be ordered. Again, malignant melanoma will yield a characteristic series of photos in 85% of all cases.[31]

5. Finally, if the diagnosis is still not clear, the *radioactive P_{32} uptake test* should be performed. The test is done in the operating room after

systemic administration of radioactive P_{32}. The procedure involves placing a radiosensitive probe through a conjunctival incision over the scleral side of the lesion. If the lesion is larger than 2.5 mm, and if the test is performed by an expert, the test has an accuracy of better than 95%.[31]

Treatment. Since the lesion is potentially lethal, the safest and most frequently used form of treatment is, at present, enucleation. Enucleation of an eye with useful vision does, however, produce functional disability and psychologic trauma, and it may involve operative morbidity. To help solve this dilemma, two other factors—tumor size and patient's age and health—should be evaluated.

Tumors are measured ophthalmoscopically using the optic nerve (2 mm at its widest diameter) as a reference.

For prognostic purposes, melanomas are classified as small if they are less than 10 mm in diameter, and as large if they are greater than 10 mm. Although all of the factors involved in tumor growth have not been elucidated, it appears that if a tumor is small when first seen, one of two natural processes may be taking place. Either the tumor has a low malignant potential and has been the same size for a long time (contained by body defenses), or it is becoming a larger and potentially lethal tumor. This hypothesis seems confirmed by the fact that enucleation of eyes with small choroidal melanomas yields the very high 5-year survival rate of 90%, whereas enucleation of eyes with small tumors showing evidence of extension through Bruch's membrane yields a 5-year survival rate of 65%.[33] Therefore, it has been suggested that when a tumor under 10 mm is initially diagnosed, it should simply be observed every 4 months. If the tumor shows any sign of growth, the eye should be enucleated.[34] On the other hand, large tumors have already demonstrated growth potential and may have already metastasized. The overall 5-year survival in patients with large melanomas treated with enucleation is 70% if there is no evidence of extension, and only about 20% if the tumor is heavily pigmented and extending through Bruch's membrane.[33] Of course, the decision to enucleate is mandatory if the eye becomes blind and painful.

The course of treatment for a malignant melanoma must be influenced by the patient's life expectancy. Thus, elderly patients with a small tumor who are in good health should be evaluated in the same way as younger patients. Elderly patients who are in poor health, on the other hand, or who are very old, may gain very little time from the enucleation of an eye with a tumor. Finally, healthy, elderly patients with a large pigmented tumor and evidence of extension may have little to gain from enucleation.

Tumor Histology and Life Expectancy. Histologically, choroidal melanomas are classified according to the predominating cell type. Both large and small tumors with spindle cells have a relatively benign prognosis, with an overall 5-year survival of 80%. Those tumors with epithelioid cells have a poor prognosis, and highly pigmented tumors with epithelioid cells have only about a 20% 5-year survival rate.[33,35]

References

1. Vaughn HG, Schlimmel H: Feasibility of electrocortical visual prostheses. In: *Visual Prosthesis, the Interdisciplinary Dialogue, Proceedings,* 2d ed. Edited by TD Sterling, EA Bering, et al. New York, Academic Press, 1971, p 144

2. Altman PL, Ditmer DS: *Metabolism.* Bethesda, Md, Fed Am Soc Exp Biol, 1968, p 391

3. Friedman E, Kopald HH, Smith TH: Retinal and choroidal blood flow determined with krypton 85 in anesthetized animals. Invest Ophthalmol 3:539, 1961

4. Wise G, Wangvivat Y: The exaggerated macular response to retinal disease. Am J Ophthalmol 61:1359, 1966

5. Flocks M, Miller J, Chao P: Retinal circulation time with the aid of fundus cinephotography. Am J Ophthalmol 48:3, 1959

6. McLean AL, Maumanee AE: Hemangioma of the choroid. Am J Ophthalmol 50:10, 1960

7. Novotny HR, Alvis DL: Method of photographing fluorescein in circulating blood in human retinal circulation. Circulation 24:82, 1961

8. Young P: Diabetes: a deadly disease on the increase. National Observer, Dec. 20, 1975, p 4

9. Ashton M: Oxygen and the growth and development of retinal vessels. In vivo and in vitro studies. Am J Ophthalmol 62:412, 1966

10. Henkind P, Wise GN: Retinal neovascularization, collaterals and vascular shunts. Br J Ophthalmol 58:413, 1974

11. Scott DJ, Dollery CT, Hill DW, et al: Fluorescein studies of diabetic retinopathy. Br Med J 1:811, 1964

12. Aiello LM, Beetham WD, Balodimas MC, et al: Ruby laser photocoagulation of diabetic proliferative retinopathy: preliminary report. In: *Symposium on Treatment of Diabetic Retinopathy.* Edited by MF Goldberg, SL Fine. Arlington, Va, DHEW, 1968, pp 437–463

13. Diabetic Retinopathy Research Group: Preliminary report of the effects of photocoagulation. Am J Ophthalmol 81:383, 1976

14. Duke-Elder S: *System of Ophthalmology,* Vol X. *Diseases of the Retina.* St. Louis, Mosby, 1967, p 582

15. Sichel J: Mémoire sur le glaucome; deuxieme partie, XIII. L'hydropisie sous choroidienne. Ann Oculist 5:243, 1841

16. De Wecker L, De Jaeger E: Traité des maladies du fond de l'oeil et atlas d'ophthalmolscopie. Paris, Adrien Delaheye, 1870

17. Leber T: Über die Entstehung der Netzhautablösung. Versammlung Ophthalmol Ges 14:18, 1882

18. Leber T: Über die Entstehung der Netzhautablösung. Versammlung Ophthalmol Ges 35:120, 1908

19. Gonin J: Pathogénie et anatomie pathologique des décollements rétiniens. Bull Soc Ophthalmol Fr 33:2, 1920

20. Delaney WY, Oates RP: Retinal detachment in the second eye. Arch Ophthalmol 96:629, 1978

21. Schepens CL, Okamura ID, Brockhurts RJ: The scleral buckling procedures. I. Surgical techniques and management. Arch Ophthalmol 58:797, 1957

22. Duke-Elder: p 797

23. Av-Shalom A, Berson D, Gombos GM: Some comments on the incidence of idiopathic retinal detachment among Africans. Am J Ophthalmol 64:384, 1967

24. Weiss H, Tassman WS: Rhegmatogenous retinal detachments in blacks. Ann Ophthalmol 10:150, 1978

25. Kansk JJ: Complications of acute posterior vitreous detachment. Am J Ophthalmol 80:44, 1975

26. Kornzweig AL: Modern concepts of senile macular degeneration. J Am Geriatr Soc 22:246, 1974

27. Sark SH: New vessel formation beneath the retinal pigment epithelium in senile eyes. Br J Ophthalmol 57:951–965, 1973

28. Duke-Elder: p 672

29. Wilkes SR, Robertson DM, Kurland L, et al: Incidence: uveal malignant melanoma in Rochester and Olmsted County, Minnesota. Paper presented at ARVO, Sarasota, Fla, 1978

30. Abramson DH, Ellsworth RM, Zimmerman LE: Monocular cancer in

retinoblastoma survivors. Trans Am Acad Ophthalmol Otolaryngol 81:OP454, 1976

31. Shields JA: Review: current approaches to the diagnosis and management of choroidal melanomas. Surv Ophthalmol 21:443, 1977

32. Coleman DJ: Ultrasonic diagnosis of tumors of the choroid. Arch Ophthalmol 91:344, 1974

33. Shammas HF, Blodi FC: Prognostic factors in choroidal and ciliary body melanomas. Arch Ophthalmol 83:27, 1970

34. Char DW: The management of small choroidal melanomas. Surv Ophthalmol 22:377, 1978

35. McLean IW, Foster WD, Zimmerman LE: Prognostic factors in small malignant melanomas of choroid and ciliary body. Arch Ophthalmol 95:48, 1977

Chapter 12

Uveitis

As with many poorly understood medical conditions, many unique descriptive terms are used in connection with uveitis. These terms are defined below:

IRITIS: Inflammation of the iris. A condition marked by ocular pain, redness, photophobia, and pupillary contraction.

IRIDOCYCLITIS: Inflammation of the iris and ciliary body. Symptoms are similar to those of iritis.

ANTERIOR UVEITIS: Another term for either iritis or iridocyclitis.

POSTERIOR UVEITIS: An inflammation of the choroid and often of the overlying retina.

CHORIORETINITIS: Another term for posterior uveitis.

GENERALIZED UVEITIS: A combination of anterior and posterior uveitis.

PANUVEITIS: Generalized uveitis.

KERATITIC PRECIPITATES (KPs): Clumps of inflammatory cells that are deposited on the back of the cornea during an attack of anterior uveitis.

GRANULOMATOUS UVEITIS: A type of uveitis in which the keratitic precipitates are large and shiny and made up of epithelioid cells and macrophages. This type of uveitis is often associated with bacterial, fungal, or parasitic infection elsewhere in the body.

NONGRANULOMATOUS UVEITIS: A type of uveitis in which the keratitic precipitates are dustlike, being made up of lymphocytes and plasma cells. This type of uveitis is considered to be associated with physical, toxic, allergenic, and viral agents.

PARSPLANITIS: Inflammation of the paraplana (a type of posterior uveitis).

CILIARY FLUSH: Dilation of the small blood vessels surrounding the limbus, yielding a red-violet perilimbal halo.

FLARE AND CELLS: Inflammation of the iris and ciliary body leading to vasodilation and increased vascular permeability of these structures. Increased amounts of protein leaking into the anterior chamber produce the "flashlight-beam-in-the-dusty-attic effect" when observed with the narrow beam of the slit lamp. This is called flare. If cells also leak into the anterior chamber, they appear as gray flecks within the beam. The intensity of the cells and flare is usually graded from 1+ to 4+.

The *uvea* of the eye is composed of the iris, ciliary body, and choroid. One look at its morphology (Fig. 12-1) will convince the reader that it is virtually a solid sheet of blood vessels, with nerves, connective tissue, muscle, and pigment filling in the spaces and pigmented epithelium coating most of its inner surface. A tissue as vascular as the uvea is much like an airline terminal; sooner or later just about everybody, or everything, passes through. Because of its vascularity, the uvea is subject to invasion by innumerable infectious agents—in fact, most bacteria, spirochetes, various rickettsiae, fungi, viruses, and a handful of protozoans have all been reported to be causes of uveitis. This apparent vulnerability to infectious agents may prompt the student to ask what the mechanisms are that normally prevent infection and inflammation, and under what conditions these mechanisms are inadequate or defective.

Causes

There are some clues to these defensive mechanisms. For example, the major inflammatory cells found in most cases of uveitis are lymphocytes, plasma cells, and epithelioid cells.[1] Infectious agents are rarely isolated in cases of uveitis, and most cases of uveitis respond to corticosteroid therapy. Finally, uveitis is often associated with ankylosing spondylitis, colitic arthritis, and Reiter's syndrome, all of which have strong immunologic features.

Thus, one must entertain the suspicion that if a section of the uveal vascular net becomes leaky (through local injury or through faulty repair and maintenance) at the same time that a potent agent is present in the capillaries, the agent may escape the pores of the vessel, complex with a uveal protein, and produce a local immune reaction.

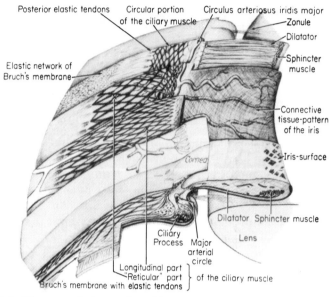

Posterior elastic tendons   Circular portion   Circulus arteriosus iridis major
of the ciliary muscle   Zonule
Dilatator
Elastic network of   Sphincter
Bruch's membrane   muscle
Connective
tissue-pattern
of the iris
Iris-surface
Cornea
Dilatator Sphincter muscle
Ciliary
Process   Major   Lens
arterial
circle
Longitudinal part
"Reticular" part   of the ciliary muscle
Bruch's membrane with elastic tendons

Figure 12-1. Diagram of the profuse blood supply to the uvea. (Reprinted with permission from Rohen JW: Vergleichende Anatomie der Retinagefässe. In: *Haut und Sinnesorgan.* Volume III, Part 4 of *Handbuch der Mikroscopischen Anatomie der Menschen.* Edited by W Moellendorff, W Bargmann. Heidelberg, Springer-Verlag, 1964, p 123.)

Uveitis may be associated with such local (i.e., eye) diseases as corneal ulcers, corneal inflammation (corneal transplant rejection, herpes zoster keratitis), leakage of lens protein (e.g., hypermature cataract), trauma (hyphema, penetrating injury), and heterochromic cyclitis (a unique type of iritis characterized by depigmentation of iris). On the other hand, uveitis is often associated with such major systemic conditions as toxoplasmosis, *Toxocara canis* infestation, tuberculosis, syphilis, viral infection, sarcoidosis, ankylosing spondylitis, Still's disease, Reiter's syndrome, and Bechet's syndrome.[2] Table 12-1 classifies these associations.

In most surveys of the etiologies of uveitis, only about a third of all cases have an identifiable cause, leaving two-thirds in the unknown-etiology ("idiopathic" or "essential") category.

Diagnosis and Treatment

A Case of Toxoplasmatic Chorioretinitis

Joan, a college freshman, complained of hazy vision in her left eye. When questioned, she stated that a similar episode 4 years before had taken 3 months to clear up. At that time her physician had treated her with "pills for an infection in her eye."

Table 12-1. Local and Systemic Conditions Associated with Uveitis

Classification	Condition
Local	Corneal ulcer
	Corneal inflammation (corneal transplant rejection, herpes zoster keratitis)
	Leakage of lens protein (e.g., hypermature cataract)
	Trauma (hyphema, penetrating injury)
	Heterochromic cyclitis (unique type of iritis characterized by depigmentation of iris)
Major systemic	*Toxoplasma gondii* infection
	Toxocara canis infestation
	Tuberculosis
	Syphilis
	Viral infection
	Sarcoidosis
	Ankylosing spondylitis
	Still's disease
	Reiter's syndrome
	Bechet's syndrome

Visual acuity was:

RE 20/20
LE 20/400

Slit-lamp examination revealed a normal anterior aspect of the eye. After pupillary dilation, the right fundus looked normal, but the left had a fluffy yellow lesion temporal to the macula (Fig. 12-2). A somewhat hazy vitreous obscured many of the fundus details, but three small pigmented areas could be seen near the fluffy lesion.

The presence of an exudative lesion near the disc, surrounded by three satellite areas of old, inactive chorioretinitis, suggested the diagnosis of recurrent toxoplasmatic chorioretinitis. Consequently, blood was drawn for a Sabin-Feldman dye test, which later proved to be positive.

Treatment. The patient was started on sulfonamide and pyrimethamine. Since the latter inhibits folic-acid synthesis, a folinic acid supplement also was prescribed. Because much of the chorioretinal reaction may be secondary to the release of long-dead encysted organisms, systemic corticosteroids were also prescribed.

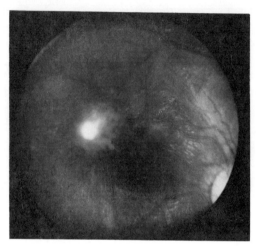

Figure 12-2. Retinal photograph showing active toxoplasmosis lesion temporal to the macula. (Reflection from the camera flash is in the center of the lesion.)

Joan's response to the medications was slow, but by the third week the vitreous had started to clear and vision in the left eye had improved to 20/100. As improvement continued, the dosages were slowly tapered. During this period, the results of the Sabin-Feldman dye test were reported, showing a titer of 1/64. After 2 months, vision was 20/20 in the left eye, the vitreous was clear, and pigment had started to surround the now-quiescent lesion.

Discussion. Toxoplasma gondii is a commonly encountered protozoan parasite often transmitted by consumption of the flesh of animals infected with the parasite in its proliferative phase, or by contact with cat feces. The initial infection in humans evokes a clinical picture of headache, fever, hepatosplenomegaly, and retinitis. In the retina, the multiplying organism destroys parasitized cells until it becomes trapped and encysted by the body's defenses. Cyst rupture may cause recurrences of the retinitis, which spreads to the choroid to produce chorioretinitis. As local capillaries dilate and become permeable in response to the inflammation, many white cells pour into the vitreous; this immigration is responsible for hazy vision—the symptom that most frequently prompts patients to seek medical care.

In about 15% of these cases of toxoplasmosis chorioretinitis, anterior uveitis also occurs. Under such circumstances, cells and flare are seen in the anterior chamber, along with a ciliary flush. Additional treatment is required to reduce the pain and photophobia of the anterior uveitis, as well as to prevent the formation of synechiae, which can either close off the filtration angle, producing glaucoma, or force the lens to stick to the pupillary border.

Diagnosis is accomplished by means of serology. The Sabin-Feldman dye-exclusion test has been largely replaced by a microtiter, indirect immunofluorescence test (which eliminates the hazard of handling live organisms associated with the dye test). Treatment is usually oral sulfonamide and pyrimethamine. If the disease progresses to anterior uveitis, local mydriatics are prescribed to keep the lens away from the pupil, and local steroids are used to quiet the inflammation. These latter two treatments are also given for uveitis arising from causes other than *Toxoplasma* infection.

References

1. Hervouet F: Pathology of endogenous uveitis. Int Ophthalmol Clin 5:713, 1965

2. Perkins ES: Uveitis survey with Institute of Ophthalmology, London. In SB Aronson: *Clinical Methods in Uveitis*. St. Louis, Mosby, 1968, pp 58–65

Chapter 13

Eye Signs and Systemic Disease

Over 150 years ago, the prominent English physician Peter Mayer Latham told his medical students, "In the eyes you will see all diseases in miniature, and you will see them as through a glass."[1] Many systemic diseases do produce eye changes—in fact, it has been suggested that of the few hundred inherited metabolic disorders, 50% produce some ocular abnormality.[2]

The purpose of this chapter is not to categorize the many ocular changes seen in systemic disease, but to discuss those systemic conditions that can be initially diagnosed by a thorough ophthalmic examination. Discussion of the diseases will be in the form of presentations of case histories, which may be categorized by the manner in which the disease may be detected ophthalmologically:

1. Diminished vision

2. Ocular irritation

3. Unusual ocular appearance

4. Routine eye examination.

The first and second categories, then, include those patients who complain of attacks of permanent or transient loss of vision, or of irritation; the third, patients who may not complain of eye problems, but whose eyes have an unusual appearance; and the fourth, patients in whom a thorough routine eye examination uncovers an early indication of a serious systemic condition. An internist faced with a perplexing case is wise to request such a routine ophthalmic examination.

Diminished Vision and Unusual Appearance

A Case of Impending Stroke

Joe was a pudgy, red-faced, balding man of 58 who enjoyed rich foods and the best wines. After his heart attack at age 55, Joe was advised to reduce his weight and to take life easy. Having just bought a motel for his oldest son, he and his son were replacing some roof shingles when Joe suddenly went blind in his left eye. As he grabbed for the railing, a feeling of light-headedness came over him. Five minutes later, Joe was back to normal, but later he decided to have his eyes checked.

Visual acuity was:

RE 20/20

LE 20/20

The ophthalmoscopic examination was normal except for the presence of glistening yellow plaques along the left superior retinal artery (Fig. 13-1). His symptoms could be explained by a cholesterol embolus from an atherosclerotic plaque in his left carotid, temporarily blocking both his retinal artery (producing the blindness) and a cerebral branch (producing the light-headedness). The refractile yellow spots in the left retina were probably cholesterol crystals known as "Hollenhorst plaques,"[3] which had broken off the carotid atherosclerotic plaques. Ophthalmodynamometry revealed diastolic pressures of 50 mmHg in the right eye, and 30 mmHg in the left eye. This finding is highly suggestive of stenosis or of plaque partially occluding the left internal carotid artery.

Treatment. The patient was sent to a neurosurgeon, and carotid angiography confirmed the diagnosis of carotid lesion.[4] The carotid plaques were removed by carotid endarterectomy and the patient has done well.

Discussion. From one-third to one-half of all strokes are caused by carotid artery disease.[5,6] In many cases, the artery is occluded by gradual fibrosis of the arterial wall. Few preliminary symptoms, caused by platelet or cholesterol emboli, announce the impending stroke. In a sense, Joe was fortunate in having an ulcerated carotid plaque; it warned him of his problem.

Several studies have shown that attacks of transient blindness in one eye *(amaurosis fugax),* together with hemispheral attacks, indicate an 80% or greater likelihood of a severe carotid lesion.[7] The presence of amaurosis fugax indicates that the following tests be performed:

1. Auscultation for neck or ocular bruit

2. Ophthalmodynamometry

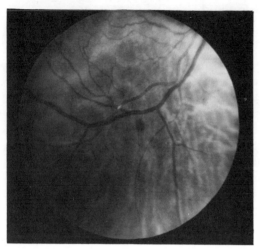

Figure 13-1. Retinal photograph showing a cholesterol embolus (Hollenhorst plaque) in the retinal artery (center of photo).

3. Evaluation of ocular fundus for
   a. attenuated arteries
   b. Hollenhorst plaques
   c. neovascularization

4. Evaluation of anterior ocular segment for
   a. unilateral arcus senilis
   b. unequal pupils
   c. neovascularization of iris
   d. Horner's syndrome

5. Noninvasive screening for carotid occlusion
   a. neurologic evaluation
   b. Doppler ultrasonography
   c. ocular plethysmography
   d. supraorbital photoplethysmography

Since carotid arteriography involves a significant risk, it should be withheld until a number of the above findings are positive.

A Case of Pituitary Tumor

Winifred was a 60-year-old woman with glaucoma that had progressed during the past few years. She had been treated for glaucoma for almost 15 years; throughout this period she continued to lose side vision, and so at different times had consulted six prominent ophthalmologists, who seemed equally divided as to the proper treatment for her glaucoma. Some suggested operation, others did not. Her medical history revealed that she was in good health, had undergone menopause early, and had lost interest in sex. Her daughter was also being treated for early glaucoma. When Winifred entered the examining room, she used her hands almost as antennae as she strode between the pieces of equipment toward the examining chair.

The results of her examination follow:

Visual acuity	RE 20/20
	LE 20/20
Pupils	Very small because of the antiglaucoma medication she was using (Carbachol, 3.0%)
Retinas	Optic nerves had cup: disc ratio of 0.6 (Fig. 13-2), which was not consistent with severe, long-standing glaucoma. The retina was otherwise normal.
Intraocular pressure	23 mmHg in each eye
Visual field	Marked constriction with only a 5° tunnel of vision remaining in each eye (Fig. 13-3).

The appearance of the optic nerves was not consistent with the constricted visual fields, and the mild glaucoma could not account for such a severe loss of peripheral vision. Such visual fields are known to occur in retinitis pigmentosa, but Winifred's retinas looked normal. The psychiatric condition hysteria might have been responsible for this picture, but Winifred definitely had the bruises to prove that she had no side vision. (For some reason, hysterically blind patients always manage to avoid objects in their path.) Could she have a pituitary tumor that had slowly grown during the last 15 years, progressively destroying the visual fibers at the optic chiasm? The history of early menopause and frigidity tended to suggest the diagnosis of chromophobic adenoma of the pituitary gland.

Treatment. The patient was referred to a neurologist who ordered endocrine studies and an x-ray of the skull. Although the endocrine studies were normal, the x-ray showed an enlargement of the sella (Fig. 13-4). The patient was referred to a neurosurgeon who successfully removed the pituitary tumor.

Discussion. Most patients with pituitary tumors initially consult their internist because of an endocrine-related disturbance. There are three

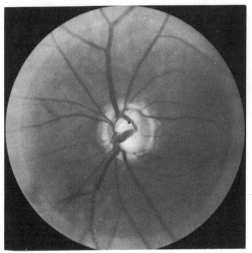

Figure 13-2. Photograph of the optic nerve showing a cup:disc ratio of 0.6. (Photographer: P. O'Connor.)

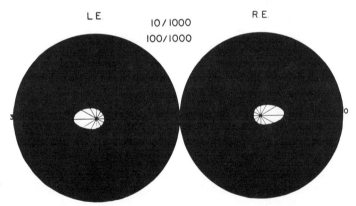

Figure 13-3. The visual field for each eye of a patient with tunnel vision.

major types of pituitary tumor. *Acidophilic adenomas* produce increased levels of growth hormone, inducing either gigantism or acromegaly. *Basophilic adenomas* induce hyperadrenalism with the attendant hypertension, diabetes, hirsutism, and the like. *Chromophobic adenomas* produce either little endocrine change or catastrophic panhypopituitarism. Of all the types of pituitary tumors, the chromophobic adenoma characteristically produces a methodic destruction of side vision *(bitemporal hemianopia)*.[7] Unfortunately, in Winifred's case the decrease in side vision had been erroneously ascribed to the glaucoma and was now irreversible.

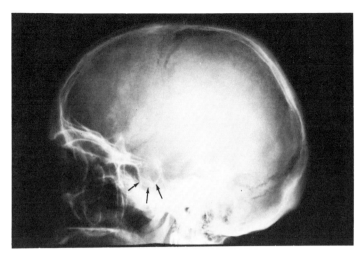

Figure 13-4. Skull x-ray illustrating an abnormal enlargement of the sella turcica indicating the presence of a pituitary tumor. Note the double floor indicating asymmetric enlargement of the gland. (Courtesy of Dr. F. Hall.)

A Case of Optic Neuritis

Ted, a 36-year-old dentist, had originally been prescribed glasses during his dental school days. Three years ago he complained of decreased vision in his right eye. At that time his right optic nerve showed the signs typical of optic neuritis. The right visual field was normal peripherally, but displayed a central 10° blind area *(central scotoma)*. The condition did not change for six weeks, at which time he was given systemic corticosteroids. His vision returned within two weeks, after which the steroids were gradually reduced to none. Then Ted reported a recurrence of the blurred vision, and this time he also noticed pain when he moved his eyes up or down.

The results of the examination follow:

Visual acuity	RE 20/400 LE 20/20
Retinas	The right optic nerve had indistinct fluffy margins, a rosy color, and an occasional hemorrhage near the disc (Fig. 13-5).
Pupillary reaction	Positive Marcus Gunn reaction on the right (i.e., the pupil dilated when a flashlight was moved

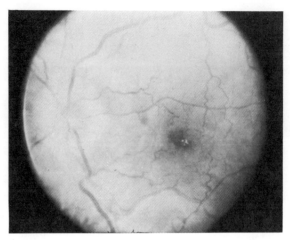

Figure 13-5. Photograph of an optic nerve displaying optic neuritis. Note the indistinct borders of the disc. (Courtesy of Dr. E. Ryan.)

Pupillary reaction
(continued)

briskly from one eye to the other and back; the illuminated pupil normally constricts or remains the same, and dilation indicates that a significant portion of the optic nerve is not functioning). Positive Marcus Gunn reactions are seen in optic neuritis, retrobulbar neuritis, optic atrophy, and advanced glaucomatous atrophy, among others.

Visual field

Right eye also displayed a central scotoma (Fig. 13-6).

Treatment. Ted was referred to a neurologist who detected a slight weakness in Ted's left hand. Spinal-fluid analysis showed abnormal amounts of gamma globulin and confirmed the diagnosis of multiple

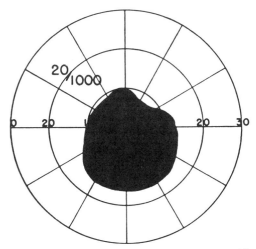

Figure 13-6. The visual field (right eye) of a patient with a 10° central scotoma.

sclerosis. The neurologist explained the diagnosis to Ted and described the disease in bold terms.

Discussion. Optic neuritis is an easy diagnosis to make once the head of the optic nerve is visualized. On occasion, however, the inflammatory process strikes not the part of the optic nerve seen with the ophthalmoscope, but, rather, the orbital portion. The diagnosis is then known as retrobulbar neuritis, a condition ironically and euphemistically described as one in which the patient sees nothing and the doctor also sees nothing. The two conditions have similar courses, and often result from viral disease, exposure to toxic chemicals, or arteriosclerotic disease. About one-half of the cases of optic neuritis are, however, associated with multiple sclerosis.[8] An early detection of the presence of multiple sclerosis, and knowledge of its characteristic history, will help the patient to plan the rest of his life in more realistic terms. Ted, for instance, took an associate into his practice, but otherwise changed his lifestyle only minimally.

A Case of Giant-Cell Arteritis

Margaret, a 70-year-old woman, told her son one morning that she could not see out of her right eye. Frail and gray-haired, she leaned heavily on her son's arm as she arrived for an appointment that same day. She had not been feeling well lately, and was suffering from an "awful" pain along the side of her head radiating to her jaw.

Visual acuity was:

RE counting fingers
LE 20/30

The ophthalmoscopic examination was within normal limits for both eyes. The area of the head along the right temple was tender to the touch. A cordlike structure (sclerotic blood vessel) could be felt with the fingers in the temporal region.

Because of the patient's age, sex, symptom of sudden blindness, and tenderness of the temporal area, the diagnosis of giant-cell arteritis was highly probable. The presence of headache and malaise suggests a systemic component of the condition and supports the diagnosis of giant-cell arteritis. An erythrocyte sedimentation rate (ESR) of 75 mm/hr (a high rate) was reported, which also is typical of the condition.

Treatment. When this disease leads to a sudden loss of vision in one eye, the case is a medical emergency. High doses of corticosteroids must be started immediately, to prevent a similar occurrence in the normal eye, and continued until the ESR returns to normal. Periodic ESR determinations are an excellent way to monitor the course of the disease.

A biopsy of the right temporal artery was performed a week after onset, and the pathologist's report confirmed the diagnosis: giant cells in the wall of the artery, destruction of the elastic tissue in the vessel wall, and intimal proliferation leading to occlusion and thrombosis. Since the disease might affect other major arteries of the body, the patient was referred to an internist.

Discussion. Giant-cell arteritis, also known as temporal arteritis, is a vicious disease that, in half of the cases, results in blindness in one or both eyes due to ischemic optic neuropathy. If untreated, its course is only weeks to months; then it remits spontaneously, leaving permanent damage in its wake.[9] The cause of the condition is unknown, but the pathologic picture and its ready response to steroids suggest an immunologic basis.

A Case of Ophthalmic Migraine

Mary, a 38-year-old housewife, had suffered a number of episodes of decreased vision in the last year. Each episode opened with flashing lights, whereupon all the vision of the left side would become hazy. She could see objects on the left, but they appeared as if through a fog. After about 20 minutes, her vision returned to normal, but she was left with a severe left-sided headache that seemed to stay the entire day. None of the over-the-counter analgesics seemed to help, and Mary usually found relief by lying down in a darkened room. Under more intense questioning, Mary remembered that the attacks started when the dosage of her contraceptive pill had been changed. She also noted that the attacks had been more frequent lately, and hypothesized that this might be due to her recent separation from her husband. Visual acuity was:

RE 20/20
LE 20/20

Ophthalmoscopic examination revealed no abnormality. Her case is representative of a migraine headache with a strong visual component. The visual complaints, which range from seeing flashing lights to a total hemianopia, are short-lived and are often, but not always, followed by a headache.

Treatment. If the episodes of the migraine are frequent and annoying enough, as was the case with Mary, the patient should be sent to an internist or neurologist. The consultant probably will place the patient on a prophylactic ergot-type medication (e.g., ergotamine), which should prevent subsequent attacks.

Discussion. Although the complete mechanism of the disease is not understood, it is felt that some substance, probably associated with the female hormones, is activated by psychologic stress. The initiating substance produces a spasm of the arteries supplying the visual cortex.[10,11] This spasm, responsible for a temporary compromise to the circulation of the region, produces the visual changes. Later, the spastic vessels overdilate, stretching the nerves that ride within the blood vessel walls and thereby causing the headache. The prophylactic medication, if taken at the first visual symptom, prevents the stage of vasodilation and pain.

A Case of Diabetes Mellitus

Carol was an agitated, somewhat thin, 35-year-old computer programmer who had had her glasses changed three times in the last six months by three different doctors and who still could not see clearly. Each new pair of glasses had allowed her to see clearly for a short while, "but only for a while." When questioned about her general health, she admitted to being excessively thirsty, always tired, and continually hungry. She quickly added, however, that those changes were probably the result of certain new job responsibilities.

The results of her examination follow:

Visual acuity   RE 20/40
                                  LE 20/40

| Refraction | By adding a small amount of minus-lens power, she was able to see the 20/20 line. |
| Ophthalmoscopy | Essentially normal except for an occasional and very small dot hemorrhage in each retina. |

The combination of thirst, weight loss, increased appetite, and frequent changes in refraction strongly suggested the diagnosis of diabetes mellitus.

Treatment. The condition was completely explained to Carol, and she was referred to an internist. Blood tests showed a blood glucose level of 300 mg/dl, with sugar and ketones in the urine. A schedule of insulin was started. When Carol's diabetes was stabilized, she was able to see clearly with her original pair of glasses.

Discussion. Table 13-1 lists the clinically significant ocular manifestations of diabetes. It has been claimed that refractive changes occur as an initial symptom of diabetes in about one-third of cases.[12] Changes of 1 D to 8 D have been reported. Apparently, a rapid and large shift in blood glucose raises the concentration of glucose in the aqueous, and, subsequently, inside the lens. Since insulin is not needed for glucose to enter lens tissue, glucose diffuses into the lens, where, some investigators believe, the enzyme aldose reductase catalyzes the conversion of glucose to sorbitol, a sugar alcohol that cannot easily diffuse out of lens tissue.[13] Accumulation of sorbitol increases intralenticular osmolarity and causes intralenticular swelling. If the new fluid lodges in the lens cortex, the converging power of the cortex decreases and the patient becomes hyperopic. If the new fluid seeps into the whole lens uniformly, ballooning its shape, the total effect is to increase the converging power and to produce myopia. This increased sensitivity of the eye lens to changes in body glucose may also explain the higher incidence of cataract formation in diabetics.

A Case of Hypertension

William, a 41-year-old black construction worker, suddenly lost vision in his right eye; if he closed his good left eye, everything was blurred and appeared dark red. A big, muscular man, William appeared superficially to be in excellent health, but he admitted that he had been suffering from headaches and that he took Alka-Seltzer regularly. His family history revealed that his mother had died of a stroke in her early forties.

Table 13-1. Clinically Significant Ocular Manifestations of Diabetes

Item Examined	Clinical Manifestations
Lids	Xanthomata of lids twice as common in diabetic population as opposed to normal population.
Iris	Neovascularization of iris, which usually progresses to the angle, producing neovascular or hemorrhagic glaucoma. This condition usually develops after diabetes of long duration and is usually preceded by severe retinopathy.
Cranial nerves	In order of frequency, 6th nerve, 3d nerve, and then 4th cranial nerve may develop vascular lesion leading to nonpermanent palsy of related extraocular muscle.
Lens	(1) There is a marked weakness in accommodation in 20% of diabetic patients, necessitating reading glasses at a younger age. (2) Transitory refractive changes may occur in diabetic patients, particularly when the blood glucose is out of control. (3) The incidence of cataracts is much higher in the diabetic population than in the normal population.
Intraocular pressure	(1) During episodes of diabetic ketosis, metabolic acidosis, and blood hyperosmolarity lead to very low intraocular pressure. (2) The diabetic population has an incidence of open-angle glaucoma higher than that of the normal population.
Retina	The incidence of diabetic retinopathy increases with the duration of the disease. Thus, 80% of patients with a 20-year history of diabetes have some form of retinopathy.

Visual acuity was:

RE counting fingers
LE 20/20

Ophthalmoscopy of the right retina showed swelling of the optic nerve (papilledema), many flame-shaped hemorrhages (one covering the macula), and a number of soft yellow exudates scattered about. The left eye showed a milder version of the same pattern, but because there were fewer hemorrhages and exudates, its arteries and veins could be studied more easily. The arteries were thin, and the veins slightly engorged, with sections of the veins compressed by the overlying arteries (A-V nicking) (Fig. 13-7).

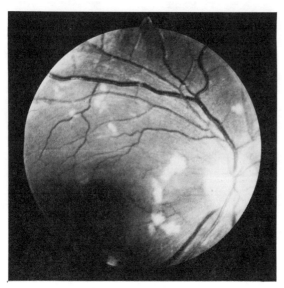

Figure 13-7. Photograph of a retina with advanced hypertensive retinopathy. Aside from the hemorrhages and exudates, note the narrowing of the arterioles and the apparent nicking of the vein by the overlying artery. (Courtesy of Dr. E. Ryan.)

William was apparently the victim of severe, probably malignant, hypertensive disease.

Treatment. William was immediately sent to an internist. On the proper antihypertensive regimen, the patient's blood pressure fell from its original 240/140 to normal, and within a month the papilledema had resolved, the hemorrhages had practically disappeared, and the patient's vision had markedly improved.

Discussion. The fundamental process involved in the retinal vessels in hypertension is vasoconstriction (often seen as segmental arterial constrictions). As more vessels go into spasm, the constricted arteries deliver less nutrition to the dependent retina and optic nerve, and areas of infarcted retina develop. When the normally transparent retina becomes infarcted, it takes on fluid, loses its transparency, and appears as a fluffy yellow exudate. Hemorrhages represent blood leaking from the capillaries, the walls of which have partially necrosed. With time, if the condition is not treated, the spastic constriction encases into a permanent structural change.

A Case of Thyroid Exophthalmos

Harriet, a woman 51 years of age, had a protrusion and redness of her eyes that gave her a truly wild-eyed appearance (Fig. 13-8). Her major

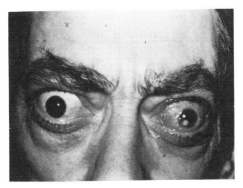

Figure 13-8. The typical appearance of a thyroid exophthalmos. Note the exposure of a corneal ulcer on the right eye.

complaint was a burning sensation in her eyes. Upon questioning, she said that she had had an episode of double vision a year ago, but was not troubled by it any longer.

The results of her examination follow:

Visual acuity	RE 20/30 LE 20/25
Exophthalmometry	RE 25 mm at 102 mm LE 23 mm
Lids	Slight cystic swelling of all lids. When the patient looked down, sclera showed between the lid margins and the limbus ("lid lag").
Conjunctiva	Inflamed, with many prominent, engorged, purple, twisting vessels present.
Cornea	Dry lesions in the inferior portion of both corneas (exposure Keratopathy) (inferior scar on right).
Eye movement	Slightly restricted in the up-and-down direction.
Ophthalmoscopy exam	Normal in both eyes.

The combination of bulging, red eyes, exposure keratopathy, lid swelling, and extraocular muscle weakness suggested the diagnosis of thyroid exophthalmos.

Treatment. The patient was sent to an internist for a thyroid evaluation. All thyroid-function studies were normal. Treatment consisted of the frequent use of artificial tears to keep the corneas moist. If the proptosis of the eyes had progressed, surgical closure of a part of the lids *(lateral tarsorrhaphy)* or orbital decompression would have been considered. In *orbital decompression,* extra room is made for the swollen tissues by removing part of the bony orbit, allowing the eye to fall back to a more normal position. Studies demonstrate that the eyes will recede 3 to 8 mm into the orbit after transantral decompression.[14]

Discussion. In thyroid exophthalmos, the extraocular muscles become infiltrated with inflammatory cells and swell to many times their normal size. B-scan ultrasonography or CAT scanning will usually reveal the muscle enlargement in both eyes. Fat and loose connective tissues in the orbit also swell. As a result, the eyeball is pushed forward. At the same time, Müller's muscle in the upper lid is kept in a state of almost chronic contraction, exposing more of the eye, particularly when the patient looks down ("lid lag"). The mechanism behind lid lag often explains the incomplete blink of these patients. An incomplete blink usually means poor wetting of the inferior cornea, leading to exposure keratopathy. Strangely enough, the onset of exophthalmos does not always coincide with the presence of hyperthyroidism. It occasionally occurs before there is any evidence of thyroid disease, and commonly develops after the thyroid disease is treated.[15] In about 5% of these cases, the increase in orbital tissue will compress the optic nerve, producing papilledema and decreasing vision. This is an emergency situation, and massive doses of systemic corticosteroids are started at once.

Findings on Routine Examination

A Case of Subacute Bacterial Endocarditis

John, a 50-year-old bank executive, was admitted to the hospital for malaise and unexplained fever. A thorough evaluation by his internist revealed no positive findings, but it was suspected that there was malignancy somewhere in the abdominal cavity, and so exploratory surgery was scheduled. During the period of preoperative preparation, a third-year medical student was assigned to review the case, since it represented an excellent example of the limitation of conventional medical diagnosis. When the student, who had graduated from optometry school before entering medical school, looked at the patient's retina, he noticed a strange type of hemorrhage. An official ophthalmologic consultation was ordered, and the presence of a hemorrhage with a yellow center was confirmed. This hemorrhage, often termed a *Roth spot,* is seen in such diseases as leukemia, multiple myeloma, Rocky Mountain spotted fever, and subacute bacterial endocarditis. The last diagnosis was confirmed when blood cultures revealed the presence of bacteria. High doses of intravenous penicillin cured the patient.

A Case of Sjögren's Syndrome

A pale, thin 22-year-old woman named Suzy was admitted to the hospital for severe malaise, fever, and cough, which had not responded to antibiotics. Routine laboratory studies simply showed Suzy to be seriously anemic and to have an infiltrative process in her lungs. Because Suzy seemed to respond to the nonspecific benefits of a hospital admission, she became more aware of herself and started complaining of irritated eyes. An ophthalmologic consultation was called for.

The results of her examination follow:

Vision	RE 20/30
	LE 20/30
Conjunctiva	Very pale.
Schirmer tear test	Almost no output of tears.
Cornea	Drying of both lower corneas (exposure Keratopathy).
Ophthalmoscopic exam	Normal.

The decreased tear production along with the exposure keratopathy strongly suggested Sjögren's syndrome. With those findings providing a new direction, more blood tests led to a positive lupus erythematosis test and to a positive latex fixation. These findings confirmed the diagnosis of the immunologic disease Sjögren's syndrome.

Treatment. The ocular irritation, due to a decrease in tear production, is often remedied by the frequent application of artificial tears. If this course does not help, the wearing of soft contact lenses, plus the use of artificial tears, usually relieves the symptoms.

A Case of Sarcoidosis

Fredricka, a 25-year-old black woman, was admitted to the hospital with presumed tuberculosis. She had the weight loss and cough typical of tuberculosis, and had shown infiltrative lung disease and enlargement of the hilar lymph nodes. When Fredricka reported blurring vision and photophobia, her doctor asked for an ophthalmologic consultation.

The results of her examination follow:

Visual acuity	RE 20/20 LE 20/50
Cornea	Slit-lamp examination revealed small, round, gray lesions (keratitic precipitates, or KPs) on the back surface of the left cornea.
Conjunctiva	Mild inflammation in left eye.
Anterior chamber	Some inflammatory cells floating in the aqueous (as seen with slit lamp).
Iris	A few yellow nodules on the iris (as seen with slit lamp).
Vitreous	Many floating bands waving in the vitreous (as seen with slit lamp).
Ophthalmoscopy	Waxy, yellow exudates, retinal hemorrhages, and some yellow sheathing of the peripheral retinal vessels in the left retina (Fig. 13-9).

Gray precipitates on the cornea, cells floating in the anterior chamber, and iris nodules all indicate anterior uveitis. The iris nodules specifically suggest sarcoid anterior uveitis; the vitreous floaters, posterior uveitis; and the sheathed vessels (vasculitis), sarcoidosis. This combination in a black person makes the diagnosis of sarcoidosis quite probable. On rare occasions, the patient with sarcoidosis will present with upper-lid swelling caused by granulomatous enlargement of the lacrimal glands palpable just below the superior orbital rim.

Treatment. Treatment consists of topical and systemic corticosteroids.

A Case of Pseudotumor Cerebri

Arlene was a moderately overweight young woman who had been having headaches for the past three months; she resisted her doctor's idea that her headaches were due to anxiety, and so to determine whether they

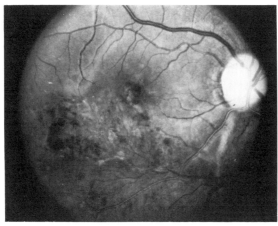

Figure 13-9. Photograph of the retina in a case of sarcoid uveitis. Note the light-colored sheathing along the vessel walls, and the intraretinal hemorrhages. (Courtesy of Dr. E. Ryan.)

could be connected with eye strain, her doctor suggested a thorough eye examination.

The results of her examination follow:

Vision	RE 20/20
	LE 20/20
Refraction	Minimal refractive error.
EOM	Full.
Fundi	The two optic nerves showed (1) increased diameter of the discs, (2) blurring of the disc margins, (3) a deep pinkness of both discs, (4) dilation of the retinal veins, (5) a few hemorrhages and a few exudates splashed around the disc edge, and (6) no spontaneous venous pulsation.

Treatment. The patient was sent to a neurologist, who could find no evidence of a brain tumor or hypertension. A spinal tap revealed an opening pressure of 350 mm H_2O. The diagnosis of pseudotumor cerebri was made and the patient responded favorably to a course of oral acetazolamide.

Discussion. The probable course of events leading to papilledema in cases of increased intracranial pressure (ICP) follows: The raised intracranial pressure is transmitted to the cerebral spinal fluid (CSF). The rise in CSF pressure is transmitted within the subarachnoid space that surrounds both optic nerves, stretching the dural sheath. The scleral tissue surrounding the optic nerve as it leaves the eye, however, does not stretch; this area acts as a tight belt around the optic nerve. Axoplasmic flow from the ganglion cells of the retina down the axons of the optic nerve is stopped at the site of the belt effect *(lamina cribrosa),* and the fibers of the optic-nerve head swell in front of the lamina cribrosa, compress the small vessels of the optic nerve head, and produce capillary and venous distention and leakage (Fig. 13-10).[16] The net effect is a nerve head that swells forward into the vitreous cavity and sideways against the retina. The swollen nerve head has a passive-hyperemia character because of the secondary venular and capillary distention.

A few clinical implications are worth noting. Papilledema usually develops within a week or two after the onset of a rise in ICP. Papilledema will usually resolve within 4 to 8 weeks after the ICP returns to normal levels. Papilledema will not develop in an atrophic optic nerve, simply because there are no axons left to swell. Although papilledema is almost always bilateral, there can be a difference in degree in the two eyes, due to variation in either the elastic capacity of each dural sheath or the point at which the subarachnoid space ends. Ophthalmoscopically, the appearance of the optic nerve in papilledema is often very similar to that of optic neuritis.

Spontaneous pulsations of the retinal veins overlying the disc appear in over 50% of the population. Studies have shown that they are absent if the CSF pressure is over 180 mm H_2O. Therefore, spontaneous venous pulsations are absent if the ICP is close to the upper limits of normal, as well as in cases of substantially elevated pressure.[17]

Papilledema usually does not interfere with visual function, but in a small percentage of cases it can lead ultimately to optic atrophy and blindness.

References

1. Bean WB: The eye: gateway to medical wisdom. In: *The Eye and Systemic Disease.* Edited by FA Mausolf. St. Louis, Mosby, 1975, p 1

2. Frederickson DS: Hereditary systemic disease of metabolism that affect the eye. In: *The Eye and Systemic Disease.* Edited by FA Mausolf. St. Louis, Mosby, 1975, pp 8–34

3. Hollenhorst RW: Significance of bright plaques in the retinal arterioles. JAMA 178:23, 1961

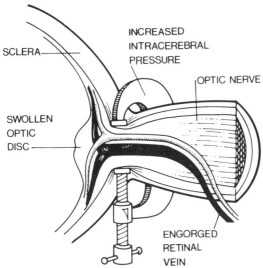

Figure 13-10. The mechanism of papilledema (see text for discussion). The clamp represents increased ICP acting at the sclera and forcing obstruction of the axoplasmic flow and venous return. (Artists: David Lobel and Laurel Cook.)

4. Pessin M, Duncan G, Mohr J, et al: Clinical and angiographic features of carotid transient ischemic attacks. N Engl J Med 296:358, 1977

5. Kannel WB, Dowber TR, Cohen ME: Vascular disease of the brain, the Framingham study. Am J Public Health 55:1355, 1965

6. Fisher CM: Anticoagulant therapy in cerebral thrombosis and cerebral embolism, a national cooperative study, interim report, part 2. Neurology (Minneap) 11:119, 1961

7. Cogan DB: *Neurology of the Visual System.* Springfield, Ill, Thomas, 1966, p 226

8. Cogan: p 179

9. Cogan: p 168

10. Symonds C: Migrainous variants. Trans Med Soc Lond 67:237, 1952

11. Mathew NT, Hrastnik F, Meyer JS: Retinal cerebral blood flow in the diagnosis of vascular headache. Headache 15:252, 1976

12. Caird FI, Pirie A, Ransell RG: *Diabetes and the Eye.* Oxford, Blackwell Scientific, 1969, pp 122–126

13. Gabbay K: Sorbitol pathway. N Engl J Med 288:16, 1973

14. Apers RG, Oosterhuis JA, Sedee E, Bierhaagh J: Results of transantral decompression in hyperthyroid exophthalmos. Document Ophthalmol 44:207, 1977

15. Forscher BK (Editor): Graves' disease. Mayo Clin Proc 47:963, 1972

16. Hayreh SS: Optic disc edema in raised intracranial pressure. Arch Ophthalmol 95:1553, 1977

17. Levin BE: The clinical significance of spontaneous pulsation of the retinal vein. Arch Neurol 35:37, 1978

Chapter 14

Ocular Pharmacology

Except for bone and cartilage, most of the tissue types in the body are present in the eyes. Consequently, the eye falls heir to many of the same diseases that afflict the other tissues. Fortunately, eye tissue also responds to many of the medications that are used to treat systemic disease. In fact, the eye sometimes is more easily treated with these medications than are other tissues, since medication may often be delivered directly to it. In this chapter, we shall discuss administration, action, indications, and contraindications of various medications.

The Prescription

Ophthalmologists, like most doctors, use a special variety of shorthand. This practice, along with the physician's less-than-perfect penmanship, often makes a prescription or an order to a nurse or pharmacist incomprehensible. A typical prescription might read:

Jones, Mary
Pilocarpine 4%
sig: OD gtt 1 q.i.d.

In simple language, Mary Jones should receive 4% pilocarpine. The prescription should be labeled (sig., *signetur* [L]: to the right eye (OD), 1 drop (gtt., *guttae* [L]; 1) four times a day (q.i.d., *quater in die* [L]). Other abbreviations important in ophthalmology are OS (left eye) and OU (both eyes).

The physician must take care that his instructions to the patient are explicit. Not long ago a patient had a piece of metal removed from his cornea in our emergency room. The doctor, expecting that the eye would begin to ache soon after the local anesthesia wore off, suggested that the patient take an aspirin if the pain became severe. The patient returned the following day with a red and angry eye. Upon examination, fragments of an aspirin tablet were found on the eye. The patient had misunderstood the doctor and had placed the aspirin on the eye in order to relieve the pain!

Routes of Administration

Drops

Most eye medications must be specially compounded to make them both water- and lipid-soluble. Only then will the drug penetrate the lipid in the corneal epithelial-cell membrane and the water in the corneal stroma, and reach the anterior chamber. Medication delivered via eyedrops will not reach the retina or choroid; thus systemic administration must be employed when these structures require medication. Because of their chemistry, topical anesthetics do not penetrate the intact cornea, iris, or ciliary body. Therefore, in preparation for an operation that will involve these structures (e.g., cataract extraction, iridectomy), the anesthetic must be either general or injected into the tissue behind the eye.

Patients often ask how many drops should be put in the eye. The average tear volume is $7 \mu l$, most of which is in the conjunctival cul-de-sac. The maximum amount of fluid that can be held by the cul-de-sac is $30 \mu l$. The average eyedrop volume is $40 \mu l$–$50 \mu l$, or a bit more than the capacity of the eye. Therefore, instillation of more than one drop at a time is unnecessary and wasteful.[1]

If the patient takes more than one type of eyedrop, he or she will often ask what the proper interval between instillations should be. Corneal penetration of most eyedrops occurs in about five minutes, and it also takes about five minutes for the tear volume to return to normal after one drop has been instilled into the eye. Therefore, an interval of five minutes is recommended between instillations.[1]

Since many medications are supplied with either a fluid, viscous, or ointment base, the patient will often ask which type is best. In a manner not completely understood, viscous and ointment vehicles deliver two to three times more active medication than saline-based preparations.[1] Ointment bases, however, often blur vision for a time, and viscous bases often leave unattrective white deposits on the lashes. Thus, the advantages and disadvantages of each mode of delivery should be considered before prescribing.

Retrobulbar Injection

To perform a retrobulbar injection, the surgeon threads the needle of the syringe along the side of the eye and then plunges the tip through the muscle cone behind the eye. It is here that an anesthetic (such as lidocaine) is injected to block the sensory impulses leaving the eye before they reach the brain and register as pain. The injection also paralyzes extraocular muscles and prevents eye movement during the surgery.

Such an injection can also be used to deliver high doses of corticosteroids to the optic nerve, retina, and choroid. In this case, the injected medication is deposited in the tissue reservoir behind the eye. The medication diffuses slowly into the blood vessels that perfuse the retina, choroid, ciliary body, iris, and anterior chamber. Although the entire body will be affected by this injection, the highest concentrations will be delivered to the eye structures.

Subconjunctival Injection

On occasion, high doses of antibiotics must be delivered to the cornea, iris, or ciliary body in order to combat a severe infection. In such instances, subconjunctival injection, i.e., injection of the antibiotic into the substance of the conjunctiva (short-circuiting the epithelial barrier of the ocular surface), delivers higher levels of the drug inside the eye than eyedrops.

Pharmacologic Agents

Mydriatics

Mydriatics are eyedrops that paralyze the iris sphincter and thus dilate or enlarge the pupil.[2] A mydriatic has three main uses:

1. To allow the doctor to see more of the retina and to see it more clearly

2. To relieve the pain often associated with pupillary spasm in corneal disease (abrasion or ulcer) or in anterior uveitis

3. To keep the pupil edge from adhering to the lens during an attack of anterior uveitis *(synechiae formation).*

Most mydriatics fall into the pharmacologic family known as parasympatholytics. They block acetylcholine action.

Mydriatics are commonly divided by their time of onset and duration of action. Naturally the times vary on an individual basis. The average times are recorded in Table 14-1.

Table 14-1. Mydriatic (Cycloplegic) Agents

Drug	Time (min) to Full Effect	Approximate Duration of Effect
Tropicamide, 0.5%	20–30	4 hr
Tropicamide, 1.0%	20–30	6 hr
Cyclopentolate, 1.0%	20–30	12 hr
Homatropine, 2.0%–5.0%	45–60	24 hr
Scopolamine, 0.3%–0.5%	45–60	48 hr
Atropine, 1.0%–4.0%	45–60	3–28 days

Anyone working in an emergency room treating corneal abrasions should commit this table to memory. I still remember the busy executive who came into the emergency room one night with a painful corneal abrasion. He made it very plain that the ocular pain did not allow him to see clearly, and that his time was worth $1,000 an hour to his company. The harried intern treated the abraded eye in the routine manner with an application of antibiotic ointment, a drop of mydriatic, an eye patch, and assurance that all would be normal in a day or two. The executive called back a week later. His eye felt better, but he still could not see with it. Upon questioning the intern, we learned that he used 4% atropine as the mydriatic. (See Table 14-1 for duration of action.) Since atropine also acts as a cycloplegic (which paralyzes accommodation), the executive could not focus clearly with that eye three weeks following his injury. The mistake was clearly an expensive one.

It is clinically observed fact that brown-eyed patients take a longer time than blue-eyed patients to achieve pupillary dilation in response to parasympatholytic mydriatics. Brown eyes also tend to remain dilated for longer periods than blue eyes. The longer duration of the mydriatic effect in the heavily pigmented iris is explained by the initial binding of the drug to the pigmented iris cells and its subsequent slow release.[3] Interestingly, the pupils of black patients frequently dilate slowly, and so they require additional instillation of the mydriatic.

The name atropine comes from Atropos, one of the three fates whose office it was to cut the thread of life. Thus, its very name puts the drug into proper perspective. The fatal dose of atropine is 1–2 g. There is enough of the drug in a 10-ml bottle of 1% solution of atropine eyedrops to kill several children if swallowed. Thus, the dangers of the drug should be stressed when prescribed.

Cycloplegics

This class of drugs includes all those that paralyze the ciliary muscle and, thus, accommodation.[2] Such a drug helps in determining the refraction of a child who continually tries to focus on everything in the examining room except the proper target. Cycloplegics are also useful in examining patients with strabismus, for it is often important to see if the amount of squint changes when all accommodation is eliminated.

Most of the drugs that paralyze the iris sphincter and produce pupillary dilation are cycloplegics (Table 14-1). The most commonly used cycloplegics are 1.0% tropicamide and 1.0% cyclopentolate. The times of onset and duration of action are similar to those for the mydriatic drugs.

Miotics

Miosis is a term that means small pupil. A miotic agent stimulates all the smooth muscles in the front of the eye. Most miotics belong to the pharmacologic family of drugs called parasympathomimetics or cholinergics, the latter term deriving from their ability to stimulate smooth muscles.

Miotics work by inducing contraction of the ciliary muscle, which pulls on the trabecular meshwork of the filtering angle and results in a greater outflow of aqueous and concomitant lowering of intraocular pressure, as well as an accommodative spasm. The second major action of the miotics is constriction of the pupil.

Glaucoma. The major indications for use of miotics in clinical ophthalmology occur in glaucoma, accommodative esotropia, and reversal of mydriasis. Miotic eyedrops are the most common treatment for glaucoma. Unhappily, along with the decreased intraocular pressure, the miotic causes pupillary constriction, which tends to dim the light from the outside world. In younger glaucoma patients with a significant amplitude of accommodation, miotics also induce a spasm of accommodation, which makes the patients nearsighted. Older patients who have lost most of their accommodation are not bothered by this action.

Accommodative Esotropia. Many patients with this type of strabismus exhibit an excess of convergence with a minimum of accommodation. In such cases, eliminating the accommodation effort with bifocals often decreases the size of the esotropia. The physician can also eliminate accommodative effort by producing a small accommodative spasm with a miotic. Drug-induced accommodation does not stimulate convergence, as does natural accommodation. Without reflex convergence, eyes tend to straighten in these patients.

Reversal of Mydriasis. The pupil is frequently dilated to allow the doctor a better view of the retina, but most mydriatics continue to affect the pupil for the remainder of the day. Can this unwanted effect be reversed quickly and easily with a miotic? The only mydriatic that can be reversed practically by pilocarpine is 10% phenylephrine. Annoying accommodative spasm, however, often outweighs the benefit of a return to normal pupil size, except in the older patient.

Miotics are often categorized as short- and long-duration.

Short Duration. Pilocarpine, 1%–4%, is the most commonly used miotic for glaucoma. Stronger concentrations are used for the more severe cases. It is usually taken four times a day.

Carbachol, 0.75%–3.0%, works in a manner similar to the action of pilocarpine. It is usually reserved for patients who are allergic to pilocarpine.

Long Duration. Echothiophate, 0.06%–0.25%, is a more potent miotic used in more severe cases of glaucoma. It has a longer duration of action and is usually taken once or twice a day. Because of its greater potency, it occasionally produces unpleasant side effects; specifically, it *may* produce diarrhea, a tingling sensation in the fingers and toes, cysts on the pupillary border, or cataracts.

Demecarium, 0.25%, is a more potent miotic similar to echothiophate, with similar attendant benefits and problems.

Inhibitors of Aqueous Secretion

As already implied, the major aim in glaucoma treatment is to improve drainage of aqueous from the eye. A second approach, which may often be used in conjunction with miotic therapy in severe cases, is the use of certain drugs to decrease the secretion of aqueous humor.

Acetazolamide. Taken by mouth, acetazolamide interferes with aqueous secretion in two ways. Since ciliary secretion depends on an enzyme called carbonic anhydrase, acetazolamide works by directly blocking this enzyme. Secondly, when this same enzyme is blocked in the kidney, the pH of the extracellular fluids turns slightly acidic, and an acidic environment also decreases ciliary-body aqueous secretion.

Epinephrine. In most branches of medicine, epinephrine is used parenterally in concentrations of 0.0001% or 0.001%. As an eyedrop, however, it is used at a 1.0% concentration in order to penetrate the eye in a significant amount. In a manner not yet understood, epinephrine decreases aqueous secretion.

Beta Blockers. These agents, useful in heart disease, can produce decreased aqueous secretion when instilled as an eyedrop.

Local Anesthetics

In a number of situations, anesthetizing the front of the eye helps both the doctor and the patient.[4] For example, the cornea must be anesthetized when performing tonometry, when removing a corneal foreign body (including sutures), and when irrigating the tear duct. The common topical or local anesthetics are chemically related to acetylcholine (ACh). In nerve tissue these agents compete with the natural ACh for the binding sites on the neuron, blocking the local action of ACh in its regulation of ion movement in the nerve fiber. The result is inability to perceive pain from the blocked area. Usually one or two drops of a topical anesthetic produce corneal anesthesia for 20–30 minutes. Proparacaine (0.5%) is the most commonly used topical corneal anesthetic. Its onset of action requires about 15 seconds, so that it is often called a miracle drug by a patient who enters the emergency room with a painful corneal foreign body. One drop of this medication stops the pain and tearing and allows the patient to open his eye so that the doctor can remove the offending agent. Tetracaine (1%) is an old favorite that is a bit more irritating than proparacaine and takes a bit longer to have an effect. Benoxinate (0.4%), a topical anesthetic similar to proparacaine, is used primarily in combination with a solution of fluorescein when performing applanation tonometry.

No discussion of ocular anesthetics would be complete without a word about mydriatics. In corneal abrasion and anterior uveitis, the pupillary sphincter often goes into spasm, which is a secondary source of pain. Cycloplegic mydriatics may be used to paralyze the sphincter. Because of its antiinflammatory action, aspirin (taken orally!) may be helpful in cases of corneal foreign body and anterior uveitis.

Corticosteroids

History. Until the early 1950s, the treatment for posterior uveitis consisted of one or two intramuscular injections of 5 million killed typhoid organisms. The injection of this foreign protein induced fever (often over 104° F), malaise, nausea, and a clearing of the uveitis. It had also been observed that another form of inflammatory disease, arthritis, often improved in women during pregnancy. To a thoughtful research pharmacologist, these two observations suggested that both arthritis and uveitis were inflammatory processes, probably caused by some toxic agent, and that there was a physiologic control activated by either pregnancy or the introduction of foreign protein that adjusted or even overrode the body's usual reaction to a damaging agent. The physiologic control turned out to be a hormone, cortisone, manufactured by the cortex of the adrenal gland. Its synthesis earned its discoverers a Nobel prize and gave mankind a very powerful medicine.[5] Since that time, the original cortisone molecule has been altered in a number of ways, so that now we have cortisonelike compounds that are more potent as antiinflammatory agents and have fewer of the undesirable side effects of cortisone. Table 14-2 compares the antiinflammatory effects of the more common corticosteroids.

Uses of Corticosteroids in Ophthalmology. A number of nonbacterial inflammations of the eye (usually allergic or viral in nature) are treated with corticosteroids.[6] In these conditions, the inflammatory response, if left untreated, may lead to permanent scarring and distortion of the delicate ocular tissue. Specific examples include the following:

1. Keratitis—induced by a virus, herpes zoster; induced by an allergic reaction to a byproduct of the tubercle bacillus known as phlyctenular keratitis; or induced by such chemical trauma as alkali splash.

2. Conjunctivitis—induced by pollen or other strong allergens.

3. Scleritis—such as that associated with arthritis.

4. Anterior uveitis—such as that associated with arthritis or sarcoidosis.

5. Posterior uveitis—induced by allergy to metabolites and cellular antigens of the toxoplasmosis parasite.

6. Optic neuritis—such as that seen in multiple sclerosis.

   In keratitis, conjunctivitis, scleritis, and anterior uveitis, the corticosteroid can be delivered in the form of eyedrops. In posterior uveitis or optic neuritis, the steroid is delivered systemically by pill or injection. A

Table 14-2. Comparison of Antiinflammatory Effects of Common Corticosteroids

Corticosteroid	Relative Strength
Cortisone	1[a]
Prednisone	5
Prednisolone	5
Methylprednisolone	6
Dexamethasone	25

[a]Weakest.

typical dose of topical steroid would be 1 or 2 drops applied to the affected eye 3 to 5 times a day (1–2 gtt t.i.d. to 5 i.d.). Another series of uses is related to the eye's overzealous response to surgical or accidental trauma. Local corticosteroids are often used after ocular surgery to whiten the inflamed eye, to decrease scar formation, and to make the eye feel less irritated.

Finally, corticosteroids are used in conjunction with corneal transplantation in an effort to block immunologic rejection.

Adverse Ocular Reactions to Corticosteroids. We have developed the idea that corticosteroids decrease the inflammatory response. Although the details of this action are not known, we do know that these agents *destroy thymocytes, slow leukocyte movement, inhibit scar formation by fibroblasts, melt away newly formed capillaries,* and *waste away muscle tissue.* Thus, it should not come as a complete surprise that prolonged use of these agents (months to years) can injure cells and confound the work of the delicate ocular tissue. Corticosteroids are a double-edged sword; they have produced many seemingly miraculous cures of eye disease, but must be administered carefully since they can incite their own brand of destructive eye disease.

Steroid glaucoma, for example, results from the prolonged use of local systemic corticosteroids, which often interferes with the efficient control of aqueous outflow and produces a progressive increase of intraocular pressure. The condition is usually reversible.

Steroid cataracts are another problem. Chronic use of systemic steroids (first noted in patients taking steroids for more than a year for severe arthritis) ultimately produces a characteristic posterior subcapsular cataract. A similar cataract is produced by high doses of ionizing radiation. Steroid cataract is not reversible in adults, but can be reversed in children.[7]

Inhibition of wound-healing results from heavy and chronic use of local steroids (e.g., as in treating a corneal transplant). Thus, sutures are not usually removed for six to nine months after a corneal transplant if high doses of steroids are used.

Infection may also follow treatment with corticosteroids. Herpes simplex virus and many fungi may incite a destructive infection in almost any part of the eye when corticosteroids are used in prolonged fashion.

Antibiotics and Antiinfective Agents

Those readers interested in statistics and trivia may be interested to know that there have been more patients treated with ocular antiinfective agents than with any other medication.[8] Almost every state requires prophylactic treatment of gonorrheal ocular infection in newborn infants;

such treatment consists of placing a drop of either 1% silver nitrate or penicillin (50,000 units/ml) in each eye.[9]

Again, for those interested in world records, *trachoma,* a chlamydial infection of the cornea, is considered to be the leading cause of blindness worldwide.[10] The agent seems to thrive where poor hygiene prevails and is rare in the Western world. Treatment consists of local and systemic *sulfonamides* or *tetracyclines.* In Tunisia, a program whereby a tube of ophthalmic tetracycline ointment can be purchased for only a few pennies without a doctor's prescription has been instrumental in significantly diminishing the incidence of the disease.

Diagnostic Methods. To diagnose a severe and potentially dangerous infection (corneal ulcer, endophthalmitis, orbital cellulitis), the basic rules for identifying a serious infection anywhere in the body obtain. Perform a smear and culture, and test for antibiotic susceptibilities of the organisms isolated. In corneal ulcer, scrape the bed of the ulcer. In endophthalmitis, tap the anterior chamber. In periorbital cellulitis, obtain a specimen from a furuncle or suppurating lesion. Immediate therapy is based on the Gram stain. If material cannot be obtained for a Gram stain, judgment must be exercised in treating for the most probable causative organism until the results of culture and susceptibility tests are obtained.

Tables 14-3 to 14-8 are intended to provide guidance in prescribing antiinfective agents. A few words of general guidance for each clinical entity may also be helpful.

Corneal Ulcers. Sight-threatening conditions can lead to perforation or scarring of the cornea. Treatment, therefore, must be aggressive. If local drops and ointment produce little improvement in 2 or 3 days, subconjunctival delivery along with topical application of the appropriate antibiotic is indicated.

Conjunctivitis. Since the concentration of antibiotics delivered to the conjunctiva is high and the inoculum is usually small, most antibiotic ointments or drops are effective, and isolation of the specific organism prior to treatment is usually not necessary.

Bacterial Endophthalmitis. A rare condition, this is seen in about one case in a thousand following intraocular surgery[11] and, more commonly, following penetrating ocular injury. Prophylactic use of chloramphenicol ointment, or some broad-spectrum combination, has drastically reduced this catastrophic postoperative complication. Treatment consists of subconjunctival and intravitreal injection of appropriate antibiotics in non-toxic concentrations.

Periorbital Cellulitis and Dacryocystitis. The venous return from the periorbital region passes through the orbit to the brain. Thus, to avoid

Table 14-3. Suspected Infectious Organism and Choice of Antiinfective Agent

Bacteria	Agent
Gram-positive cocci	
Staphylococcus sp. (penicillinase negative)	Penicillin
Streptococcus sp.	Bacitracin
Streptococcus pneumoniae	Erythromycin
	Ampicillin
	Neomycin
	Lincomycin
	Gentamycin
Penicillinase-producing Staphylococcus sp.	Nafcillin
	Methicillin
	Vancomycin
	Cephalosporin
	Dicloxacillin
Gram-negative bacilli	
Pseudomonas sp.	Polymyxin B
	Colistin
	Gentamycin
	Chloramphenicol
Proteus sp.	Neomycin
Escherichia coli	Chloramphenicol
Klebsiella pneumoniae	Streptomycin
	Gentamycin
	Polymyxin B (not effective against Proteus)
Gram-negative cocci	
Neisseria gonorrhoeae	Penicillin
	Chloramphenicol
	Tetracycline
	Gentamycin
	Neomycin
	Bacitracin

conditions such as cavernous sinus thrombosis, treatment should be started immediately. The most common causative agent in these periorbital infections is *Staphylococcus aureus.*

Ocular Side Effects of Systemic Drugs

Not long ago an internist was asked to examine a young woman who was being considered for a very responsible job in a large insurance company.

Table 14-4. Agents Used in Treating Conjunctivitis

Nature of Infection	Agent		Concentration	Dose
Bacterial	Combination drops	Polymyxin B	2.5 mg/ml	q.i.d.
		Neomycin	1.75 mg/ml	q.i.d.
		Gramicidin	0.025 mg/ml	q.i.d.
	Sulfacetamide drops		30% solution	q.i.d.
	Sulfasoxazole drops		4% solution	q.i.d.
	Combination ointment	Polymyxin B	500 U/g	t.i.d.
		Bacitracin	400 U/g	t.i.d.
		Neomycin	3.5 mg/g	t.i.d.
	Erythromycin ointment		0.5% (5 mg/g)	t.i.d.
Chlamydial	Tetracycline tablets		250 mg	q.i.d. (28 days)
	Tetracycline ointment		0.5% or 1.0%	t.i.d. (28 days)

Table 14-5. Agents Used in Treating Corneal Ulcers

Nature of Infection	Agent	Concentration	Route	Dosage
Bacterial	Gentamycin	1% 20 mg	drops subconjunctival injection	q.i.d.–5 i.d. q.d. × 3
	Chloramphenicol	0.5% 1.0% 1.25 mg	drops ointment subconjunctival injection	q.i.d.–5 i.d. q.i.d. q.i.d.
	Neosporin		drops ointment	q.i.d.–5 i.d. q.i.d.
	Colistin	0.12%	drops subconjunctival injection	5 i.d. q.i.d.
Viral	Idoxuridine (IDU)	0.1% 0.5%	drops ointment	5 i.d. 5 i.d.
	Adenine Arabinoside (ARA-A)	3.0%	ointment	5 i.d.
Fungal	Pimaricin	5.0%	drops	q2h
	Nystatin cream	100,000 U/g	drops	q2h

Table 14-6. Agents Used in Treating Bacterial and Fungal Endophthalmitis

Nature of Infection	Type of Agent	Agent	Route	Dosage
Bacterial—Gram-positive and Gram-negative	Systemic	Chloramphenicol	p.o., i.m., i.v.	3 g priming dose 1 g q8h
		Ampicillin	p.o.	0.5–1.0 g priming dose 0.5 g q8h
		Penicillin G plus	i.v.	20 million U/day
		Streptomycin	i.m.	1.0 g priming dose 0.5 g q8h
		Tetracycline	p.o.	1.0 g priming dose 0.5 g q6h
		Cephalothin	i.v.	2.0 g q4h × 3 days 1.0 g q4h
		Kanamycin	i.m.	0.5 g q8h
Bacterial—Gram-positive		Vancomycin	i.v.	2 g priming dose 1 g q12h
		Penicillin G	i.v.	20 million U/day
		Nafcillin	p.o.	1.0 g q6h
		Dicloxacillin	p.o.	1.0 g q6h

Chloromycetin	subconjunctival	1.25 mg/0.5 ml qd
Neomycin	subconjunctival	1.25 mg/1.5 ml qd
Penicillin	subconjunctival	25,000 U/1 ml qd
Bacitracin	subconjunctival	20 U/ml qd
Polymyxin B	subconjunctival	1000 U/0.5 ml qd

Table 14–7. Agents Used in Treating Bacterial Orbital Cellulitis and Dacryocystitis

Agents	Route	Dosage
Chloramphenicol	p.o., i.m., i.v.	1 g q8h
Ampicillin	p.o.	0.5 g q8h
Penicillin G	i.v.	20 million U/day
Streptomycin	p.o.	0.5 g q8h
Tetracycline	p.o.	0.5 g q6h
Cephalothin	i.v.	1.0 g q4h
Kanamycin	i.m.	0.5 g q8h
Vancomycin	i.v.	1.0 g q12h
Nafcillin	p.o.	1.0 g q6h
Dicloxacillin	p.o.	1.0 g q6h
Erythromycin	p.o.	0.5 g q6h

Table 14–8. Agents Used in Combination to Treat Toxoplasmosis Uveitis

Agent	Route	Dosage
Pyrimethamine	p.o.	200 mg/day for 2 days 25 mg b.i.d.
Sulfadiazine	p.o.	1 g q.i.d.
Folinic acid	p.o.	5 g t.i.d.
Prednisone	p.o.	60 mg q.o.d.

Upon questioning, she reported that her medical and psychologic history had been without incident. Her physical examination findings also were normal, with one small exception. The internist noted an odd dark spot on the lens of each eye and called me for consultation. The spot on the lens was a yellow-brown deposit of pigment seen only in patients who have been receiving large doses of the tranquilizer chlorpromazine for a few years. Invariably, these patients have been in mental hospitals while taking these high doses of the drug. That astute observation by the internist saved the woman and the company much grief.

The story illustrates that medications used to treat systemic disease may affect the eye.[12] In this section, these drugs are categorized according to the changes they can produce in the eye.

Decreasing Vision

Chloroquine. This drug, developed primarily to treat malaria, now has its greatest use in treating such collagen-vascular diseases as rheumatoid arthritis. If taken for long periods in high doses, the drug can cause a pigmentary degeneration of the macula. It is rare to see a case of chloroquine retinopathy in which the cumulative dose over a few years was less than 250 g. Before the retinal changes set in, yellow-brown chloroquine deposits may be seen in the cornea and lens.

Digitalis. This most famous drug for failing hearts occasionally produces episodes of blurred vision or strangely colored vision. In a small group of patients, the drug apparently interferes with the function of the cones or rods. When the dosage is decreased, the visual problem disappears.

Ethambutol. This drug is an effective antituberculosis agent. If given in dosages over 25 mg/kg, it has been known to produce a retrobulbar neuritis. Such patients report decreased vision and often manifest problems with their color discrimination. When the drug is stopped, the vision returns to normal.[13]

Chloramphenicol. This drug is one of our most valuable allies in cases of severe systemic infection. Unfortunately, it has been known to cause optic neuritis, primarily in children. Although the basis for the toxic reaction is not clear, in one case the B-vitamins pyridoxine and cyanocobalamin reversed the neuritis while the child continued to take the chloramphenicol.[14]

Induced Myopia

Occasionally, some of the popular diuretics and their close chemical relatives induce acute, transient episodes of myopia.[15] During the ocular examination, normal vision is restored with the proper added lens. The mechanism for this acute change in refraction is thought to involve an acute swelling of the lens of the eye. The agents that have been reported to cause acute transient myopia include acetazolamide, sulfonamides (close chemical relatives of acetazolamide), hydrochlorothiazide, and chlorothiazide.

Cataracts

Posterior subcapsular cataract is a common complication of both local and systemic long-term corticosteroid treatment. Typically, the patient is an arthritic or asthmatic who has been taking the steroid orally for two years or longer.

Nonsymptomatic Eye Changes

During a routine eye examination the doctor may note an abnormality of which the patient is unaware but which reflects a drug-induced systemic change. These abnormalities and the drugs that cause them are discussed below.

Papilledema. Swelling of the optic nerve can be brought about by a drug-induced increase in intracranial pressure. The condition known as *pseudotumor cerebri* usually causes severe headaches, and many headache sufferers often consult an eye doctor to rule out ocular causation of their problem. Some of the more common systemic medications that have been known to produce papilledema are corticosteroids (prolonged administration, usually in children), vitamin A (in high doses), and tetracycline (often in children).

Corneal and Lens Pigmentary Deposits. Both the phenothiazines (e.g., chlorpromazine) and chloroquine can produce yellowish-brown swirls in the subepithelial zone of the cornea and lens.[16] These areas represent drug deposits that change color on prolonged exposure to light. Only those parts of the cornea not covered by the lids accumulate deposits.

Corneal Changes. Contraceptive hormones are sometimes implicated in decreased tolerence to contact lenses.[17] The mechanism of this action is not fully understood, but seems to involve increased corneal hydration or a change in tear composition.

Ocular Side Effects of Eyedrops

The eyedrops discussed in this chapter are all potent medications with complex molecular configurations. Therefore, one should expect to encounter occasional allergic or other adverse reactions when these agents are used. Below is a list of the medications that are the more frequent offenders:

1. Atropine—may produce contact dermatitis of the lids and cheek.

2. Epinephrine—reactive hyperemia (chronic red eyes are often the hallmark of patients taking epinephrine drops for glaucoma).

3. Neomycin—produces a superficial punctate keratitis in a small percentage of patients; often produces contact dermatitis.

4. Pilocarpine—most miotics produce a headache or browache during the first week of use. The ache then leaves even if the medication is continued.

Vitamins and the Eye

Many people say that eating carrots (which contain a vitamin A precursor) prevents blindness. Vitamin C eyedrops are sold throughout the world as a prophylaxis against cataract formation. Thiamine is said to reverse inflammation of the optic nerve and to cure optic atrophy. Niacin, which brings a flush to the face and increases superficial peripheral blood circulation, is advertised as a treatment for senile macular degeneration. These four claims suggest that certain degenerative eye conditions result from malnutrition of the ocular tissues. In examining the validity of these claims, it may be helpful to look at the ocular effects of unquestionable malnutrition in humans, a condition all too common during wartime and in areas of great poverty.

Vitamin A Deficiency

In 1814 an English naval surgeon named Bamfield noted that his East Indian sailors had very poor night vision. This type of night blindness often accompanied scurvy but did not improve when the sailors were fed lemon-juice supplements. The night blindness did improve, however, when the sailors were given a balanced diet.[18] In 1860, a Confederate army surgeon reported the constant failure of the pupil to constrict to the light of a single candle (a good description of night blindness) in some of his poorly fed soldiers. He attributed the condition to a meager diet, absence of vegetable oil, and the other depressing influences of a soldier's life.[18]

In all of the wartime situations noted, it was a deficiency of vitamin A that led to night blindness, corneal drying, and atrophy of the goblet cells of the conjunctiva. But conditions that interfere with the absorption of vitamin A from the intestines (celiac disease, sprue, and hepatic cirrhosis) also produce signs of vitamin A deficiency. It is only under special and severe circumstances of deficiency, however, that vitamin A prevents blindness.

Vitamin B (Thiamine, Niacin) Deficiency

During World War II, the Japanese maintained an enormous camp for Australian prisoners-of-war in Singapore.[16] The diet at the camp consisted primarily of polished rice and occasional servings of vegetable soup. This diet was low in such B-vitamins as riboflavin and thiamine. Woodruff, an Australian army surgeon who was imprisoned at the camp, in 17 months recorded 1153 cases of what he called nutritional amblyopia. On closer inspection of Woodruff's record, we can see that when the soldiers had been on such a vitamin B-deficient diet for 6 to 12 months, they developed a decrease in their central vision. Autopsy studies showed that there had been a selective atrophy of the macula fibers of the optic nerve. If the prisoners had been treated early with vitamin B supplements, the condition would have been reversible. Unhappily, most of the prisoners were on the deficient diet for such a prolonged period that central vision was lost permanently.

It seems that only under severe vitamin B restriction (thiamine probably being the key element) does a very special form of optic nerve damage take place. In 1945, Dr. Ida Mann, a famous Australian ophthalmologist, studied the incidence of different ocular diseases in various parts of the world. She examined many natives who subsisted on vitamin B-deficient diets and reported that she was struck by the rarity of eye disease related to vitamin B deficiency.

Controlled studies have further demonstrated that thiamine cannot reverse nerve degeneration (e.g., as found in multiple sclerosis); niacin does not reverse senile macular degeneration; and vitamin C does not alter cataracts.

Patient Compliance

No chapter on therapeutic drugs is really complete without a few words on how often the patient actually takes the prescribed drugs. Obviously, a brilliant diagnosis followed by an organized therapeutic regimen achieves little if the patient does not take the medicine. A number of studies have been performed on populations of ambulatory patients with renal or hypertensive disease. These patients were given medication and, unknown to them, their urine and blood were assayed for the presence of the drug. The study revealed that one-half of the patients did not take the prescribed medication.[19]

Several factors may influence patient compliance.[20] Studies have shown, first of all, that there is no correlation between intelligence and compliance. In the Vincent study of glaucoma patients, another factor, understanding of the potential blinding effect of the disease, was shown not to be significant in separating compliers from noncompliers.[21] In a study of diabetics, Watkins found that those patients with the highest cognitive knowledge of their disease also had the poorest compliance and that the longer a patient had been receiving insulin, the more likely he was to make an error in insulin dosage.[22]

Common sense suggests that the more medications a patient must keep track of, the greater the likelihood of his making a mistake. In a study of 26 elderly patients, it was noted that *all* those patients taking five or six medications a day consistently made at least one error, and that *most* patients taking three or more drugs made an error.[23]

Two hundred thirty-nine sedentary, middle-aged men, at high risk for developing coronary artery disease, were placed on a supervised physical-activity program.[24] If the wife's attitude toward participation was positive, there was 80% compliance. If the wife's attitude was neutral or negative, only 40% compliance was noted.

Schwartz studied medication errors made by elderly, chronically ill patients and showed that error-makers were more likely to be widowed, divorced, separated, or living alone.[25]

If the patient can see the same doctor at each office visit, compliance improves. Charney showed that children were more apt to take the proper number of penicillin pills when prescribed by their own physicians rather than when prescribed by the physicians' associates.[26] Finally, repeated doctor's visits also help to reinforce compliance. In following serum-diphenylhydantoin levels in a series of epileptics, therapeutic levels of the drug were noted more commonly in those patients who saw their doctors frequently and who were admonished when the serum levels fell.[27]

References

1. Mishima S: Pharmacology of ophthalmic solutions. Med Cont Lens Bull 4:22, 1978

2. Havener WH: *Ocular Pharmacology.* St. Louis, Mosby, 1970, p167

3. Salazar M, Shimada K, Patil PN: Iris pigmentation and atropine myhriasis. J Pharmacol Exp Ther 197:79, 1976

4. Havener: p 46

5. Goodman LS, Gilman S: *The Pharmacological Basis of Therapeutics,* 3d ed. New York, Macmillan, 1965, p 1609

6. Havener: p 274

7. Forman AR, Loreto JA, Tina LU: Reversibility of corticosteroid-associated cataracts in children with the nephrotic syndrome. Am J Ophthalmol 81:75, 1977

8. Havener: p 86

9. Havener: p 340

10. Havener: p 500

11. Allen HF, Mangiaracine AB: Bacterial endophthalmitis after cataract extraction. II. Incidence in 36,000 consecutive operations. Arch Ophthalmol 91:3, 1974

12. Grant WM: *Toxicology of the Eye.* Springfield, Ill, Thomas, 1974, p 812

13. Grant: p 459

14. Grant: p 254

15. Grant: p 31

16. Grant: p 31

17. Grant: p 309

18. MacLaren DS: *Malnutrition and the Eye.* New York, Academic Press, 1963, p 157–203

19. Lowenthal DT, Briggs WA, et al: Patient compliance for antihypertensive medication. The usefulness of urine samples. Curr Ther Res 19:405, 1976

20. Blackwell B: The drug defaulter. Clin Pharmacol Ther 13:841, 1972

21. Vincent P: Factors influencing patient non-compliance: a theoretical approach. Nurs Res 20:509, 1971

22. Watkins JD, Williams TP, Martin DA: A study of diabetic patients at home. Am J Public Health 57:452, 1967

23. Curtis EB: Medication errors made by patients. Nurs Outlook 9:290, 1960

24. Heinzelman F, Bagley R: Response to physical activity programs and their effects on health behavior. Public Health Rep 85:905, 1970

25. Schwartz D, Wang M, Zeitz L: Medication errors made by elderly, chronically ill patients. Am J Public Health 52:2018, 1962

26. Charney E, Bynum R, Eldridge D: How well do patients take oral penicillin? A collaborative study in private practice. Pediatrics 40:182, 1967

27. Lund M, Jorgensen RS, Kuhl R: Serum diphenylhydantoin in ambulant patients with epilepsy. Epilepsia (Amst) 5:51, 1964

Chapter 15

Over-the-Counter Eyedrops

Many Americans feel that certain eye conditions can be treated without the help of a doctor, which is supported by the fact that about one-third of the entire eye medication market is composed of nonprescription, over-the-counter (OTC) preparations. In 1974 sales amounted to almost $25 million.

All OTC products can be purchased without a doctor's prescription. Some are "ethically promoted" (minimally advertised to the lay public, and primarily suggested by physicians), such as Vasocon® and Prefrin®, and others are full-fledged "proprietary" drugs (advertised to the lay public), such as Visine® or Murine®.

Decongestants

A popular ocular decongestant is advertised as "getting the red out." Common causes of redness are irritants such as dirt, dust, and air pollutants; osmotic agents such as sea water, which is hypertonic, and lake and pool water, which is hypotonic; prolonged exposure to reflected ultraviolet radiation, as might result from a day on the seaside or from skiing on a snow-covered mountain; alcoholic beverages, which dilate most of the body's blood vessels; and allergens such as pollen, which cause allergic inflammation in susceptible people.

All of these irritative agents activate cells in the conjunctiva to secrete a histaminelike agent that dilates the conjunctival blood vessels. As the vessels dilate, they leak a small amount of serum that makes the conjunctiva feel swollen, heavy, and sometimes itchy or irritated. Tearing usually is the result of such stimuli.

Indications for Decongestant Use

Naturally, many serious eye diseases also present as irritated red eyes. How should the patient be advised as to when to see a doctor, and when to self-medicate with an OTC preparation? Most of the time, the patient knows when he has been in an eye-irritating environment. Sometimes, however, the cause is not apparent, and the patient may need to consult a doctor under the following circumstances:

1. If vision is impaired.

2. If the eye is painful.

3. If bright light is bothersome.

4. If the eyelids stick together.

5. If redness does not improve after use of an OTC decongestant for one to two days.

6. If a foreign body is present in the eye.

Ingredients

The active ingredient in all ocular decongestants is a class of drugs related to epinephrine, called sympathomimetics.[1] They include the following:

1. Ephedrine hydrochloride, 0.12%, which tends to be short-acting and is rarely used today.

2. Phenylephrine hydrochloride, 0.12%, which is the most commonly used ocular decongestant. Phenylephrine oxidizes and tends to lose its potency if the container is opened frequently.

3. Naphazoline hydrochloride, 0.10%, which seems to be a little less potent than phenylephrine products.

4. Tetrahydrazoline hydrochloride, 0.05%, which seems to be of potency comparable to the phenylephrine products, but which has a little greater stability.

Dangers

The label on most decongestants says "Do not use in cases of glaucoma." This is based on the knowledge that sympathomimetics not only constrict blood vessels, but also dilate the pupil. In patients with narrow-angle glaucoma, pupillary dilation can convert the narrow angle to a closed angle and precipitate a severe glaucoma attack. In reality, however, the concentration of sympathomimetic allowed in an OTC preparation is too small to affect the pupil *unless* a corneal abrasion is present (a condition that itself is very painful). When a corneal abrasion is present, a large dose of the decongestant is allowed entrance into the inside of the eye, and pupillary dilation can then occur. OTC decongestants are not contraindicated in patients with open-angle glaucoma, and are only contraindicated in people with narrow-angle glaucoma and an abraded cornea.

Artificial Tears (Eye Lotions)

The surface of the cornea is continuously moistened and cleaned by a slow but steady trickle of tears. The tears themselves are a complex mixture of the watery secretions of the lacrimal gland, the mucus secretion of the conjunctival cells, and the oily secretions of the meibomian glands of the lid. The tears, in turn, are continuously swept over the cornea by eye closures and blinks.

A deficiency of tears usually reflects a serious eye problem and should be evaluated by an ophthalmologist, as should any paralysis of eye closure. Dry eyes, however, may also be a minor problem resulting from variation in normal blink rate. When driving or reading, we concentrate more and blink less.[2] Therefore, periods of prolonged reading, studying, or driving tend to dry the corneal surface, producing a dry or irritated feeling in people with marginal wetting systems. In such situations, placing a drop of a bland, slightly viscous solution on the eye often relieves the discomfort. This class of eye preparation is known as artificial tears or eye lotions.

These clear, bland agents alter the surface tension of the natural tears and create relatively long-lasting liquid films over the ocular surface.[3] They not only moisten the ocular surface, but also decrease the friction between lid and cornea during a blink by a lubricating action. The following agents are commonly used in the various OTC artificial tear preparations.

1. Methylcellulose, 0.5% to 1%.

2. Hydroxypropylmethylcellulose, 1%.

3. Polyvinyl alcohol, 1.4%.

4. Polyvinyl pyrrolidone, 1.7%.

5. Hydroxyethylcellulose, 0.8%.

6. Absorbase.

7. Gelatin, U.S.P.

8. Propylene glycol, U.S.P.

9. Sodium carboxymethylcellulose, U.S.P.

All of these agents seem to perform satisfactorily. Continued use of the more viscous agents, however, often leads to dry, unsightly white strands along the lid margin.

Eye Washes

In general, eye washes are used primarily to irrigate an eye that has been splashed by a dangerous chemical, or to dislodge a foreign particle stuck to the surface of the eye or inner lid. They contain no active ingredients and their main prerequisite is sterility. The ingredients listed on the label usually include a preservative, buffering agents, and agents that regulate osmolarity.

If a victim of a chemical splash to the eyes comes into an emergency room, and no OTC eye wash is available, sterile saline or isotonic saline (i.v. solution) can be used for eye irrigation.

Active Ingredients of OTC Preparations

Preservatives

All commercial eye preparations are sterile when the container is closed by the manufacturer. Preservatives are in the container so that the contents will remain sterile once it is opened and used by the patient. In general, preservatives do not allow the common bacterial and fungal pathogens to grow. In the concentrations used, the preservatives do not harm the ocular tissue. Benzalkonium chloride, chlorbutanol, phenylmercuric nitrate, phenylmercuric acetate, thimerosal, methylparaben, propylparaben, and disodium ethylenediaminetetraacetate (EDTA) are some of the commonly used preservatives.

Buffers

The pH of normal tears is 7.4, and the normal eye can tolerate a pH range of 6–8 without irritation. The pH of the eyedrop must be within that range to minimize irritation. Since certain medications, such as local anesthetics and cycloplegics, decompose at neutral or alkaline pH, a buffer is added to maintain drug stability and activity.

Osmolarity

The osmolarity of tears is equivalent to that of a 0.9% (isotonic) solution of sodium chloride. Solutions that are hypotonic (tap water) or hypertonic (prescription drops such as 10% phenylephrine) are irritating and cause a burning sensation. Thus, sodium chloride or potassium chloride is often added to an OTC preparation in order to make it isotonic with natural tears.

Warnings

Eye cups should not be used, as they are an outmoded and dangerous method of delivering eye medication and may transfer infection easily from one eye to another if the cup is not properly sterilized—and it almost never is. Rosepetal water, which is mildly astringent, weakly vasoconstrictive, essentially valueless, and possibly antigenic, should be avoided. Yellow oxide of mercury should also be avoided. This old favorite initially was developed as a mild antiinfective agent for bacterial conjunctivitis. It is a combination of mercuric chloride and sodium hydroxide. Mercuric oxide as a soluble salt does have antiinfective properties; but to comply with Federal Drug Administration standards, the medication is rendered free of contamination—as well as of any antiseptic effect—by washing out the soluble mercuric oxide. What is left is a mercuric compound that, like many other mercuric compounds, is a potent allergen to some people.

Contact Lens Solutions

The contact lens is initially attractive, for it lets the patient see without those annoying glasses; but there are problems. The plastic lens repels the tear fluid. Thus the lens may rub against the cornea and grate against the inner lid during a blink. The lens may also introduce bacteria or viruses into the eye at each removal and insertion.

Wetting Agents

If a clean, dry plastic lens is dipped in water and then removed, the surface does not wet evenly; the water forms small drops on the surface. The pharmaceutical industry solved this problem by formulating the wetting solution. Rubbing the wetting agent on the lens allows the lens to wet evenly with tears; it forms a film thick enough to allow the lens to stick to the finger during insertion; and it envelops the lens in a large, viscous drop that allows the lens to almost "jump" into the eye as it is brought toward the eye.[4] Just about any of the active viscous ingredients found in artificial tears (polyvinyl alcohol, polyvinyl pyrrolidone, hydroxypropylmethylcellulose, or absorbase) will perform the above functions. As in any OTC preparation, other ingredients include a buffer, a tonicity agent, and a preservative.

Soaking Solutions

After the lens is removed, it usually is covered with mucoid secretions that tend to dry and harden on the surface. These secretions may also harbor microorganisms, which may multiply once they are taken from the naturally disinfecting devices of the eye. For these reasons, the lens should be placed in a soaking solution overnight. Interestingly, a combination of a favorite OTC preservative and detergent (benzalkonium chloride) and a solvent (chlorbutanol) effectively removes the ocular secretions, destroying organisms sequestered on the lens, and keeping the plastic from drying out.

Cleaning Solutions

In the event that wetting the lens before insertion and soaking the lens after removal do not keep the lens free of protein, oil deposits, and cosmetics, a cleaning solution may be needed. A good all-purpose household detergent would be an effective cleaning agent, but such detergents are irritating if even a small amount is left on the lens. The safer commercial contact-lens cleaning solutions, containing nonionic detergents or benzine, should be used.

Soft Contact-Lens Solutions

Since soft contact lenses have a high water content, they need no wetting agent, but they must be sterilized between wearings. To accomplish this, they are either placed in a saline solution and boiled (usually in a special automatically controlled boiling device), or put through a series of rinsings with a special disinfectant. Then they are stored in a saline solution (complete with preservatives, tonicity agents, and buffers).

Unfortunately, the boiling routine often seems to precipitate secretions and debris onto the soft surface. If this occurs, an enzymatic cleaner (containing papain) can be used to digest the debris off the lens surface.

References

1. Lofholm PW: Ophthalmic products. In: *The Handbook of Non-Prescription Drugs.* Edited by LL Hawkins. Washington, DC, American Pharmaceutical Association, 1973, pp 99–107

2. Drew GC: Variation in reflex blink rate during visual motor tasks. Q J Exp Psychol 3:73, 1951

3. Benedetto DA, Shah DO, Kaufman HE: The instilled fluid dynamics and surface chemistry of polymers in the pre-ocular tear film. Invest Ophthalmol 14:887, 1975

4. Mandell RB: *Contact-Lens Practice, Hard and Flexible Lenses.* Springfield, Ill, Thomas, 1974, pp 255–284

Chapter 16

First Aid to the Eye

Most patients with an eye problem have a subjective complaint (e.g., eye pain, blurred vision) and an objective complaint (e.g., the eye is red, has a lump, or is otherwise abnormal in appearance). The patient may also provide a helpful history (recent trauma, previous similar episode with diagnosis). With such a patient, the examiner has three basic tasks: to diagnose, to ascertain the severity of the condition, and to treat the condition.

First, make a diagnosis. As in other fields of medicine, this involves taking an adequate history and doing a thorough physical examination. Inherent in the making of a diagnosis is a knowledge of how benign or dangerous a condition may be. For example, a fist-induced "black eye" is often associated with fracture of the floor of the orbit, hemorrhage inside the eye, or tearing of the retina. Knowing the risks of a black eye puts the examiner on guard.

Second, ascertain severity. Certain tests will be required to determine the severity of the black eye. If the results of the test reveal only minor subcutaneous bleeding, the treatment may simply be cold compresses.

Third, develop a plan of treatment. If the results of the tests show more than superficial damage, however, treatment must include consultation with an ophthalmologist.

Diagnosis

The diagnostic process involved in evaluating, for example, a red, painful eye, flows like the pages of a good detective story. There are only five major diagnostic categories; i.e., the source of the pain must be in the conjunctiva, cornea, iris, anterior chamber, or sclera. Red eyes may be associated with such infrequent conditions as Bechet's disease, Reiter's syndrome, Still's disease, Cogan's syndrome, relapsing polychondritis, and gout. These conditions, however, will not be discussed in this chapter, which focuses on common disorders.

History

Since these basic categories are anatomic, Figure 16-1 is a good picture to keep in mind when evaluating a red eye. Starting an examination sometimes provides immediate clues to certain diagnoses. A few key words, such as "Eye sticks together in the morning" or "I'm worried about this painless red spot on my eye," can define the condition—in these cases, bacterial conjunctivitis and subconjunctival hemorrhage, respectively.

Examination

After the history, determine and record visual acuity. Conjunctival disease and episcleritis do not affect vision, while iritis, a central corneal ulcer, and acute glaucoma do. Further examination of an irritated eye may require a drop of local anesthetic (0.5% proparacaine) on the eye (Fig. 16-2). This will achieve three results. First, giving relief is in itself a physician's aim. Second, making the patient more comfortable will allow easier examination of the eye. Finally, persistence of pain after local anesthesia suggests that the trouble is deep in the eye, i.e., iritis or glaucoma. If the pain disappears after topical anesthesia, a diagnosis of a surface problem, such as corneal abrasion or ulcer, or conjunctivitis, is suggested.

Cornea. Examining the cornea is done best with a flashlight held at the side of the eye (Fig. 16-3). A corneal foreign body, or an ulcerated or abraded area, often appears gray against a dark background. If this test does not yield conclusive results, take a strip of sterile fluorescein paper, moisten an edge with a drop of local anesthetic or an antibiotic eyedrop, and touch the lower lid with the moistened edge. After a few blinks, the fluorescein will outline the diseased area in yellow when the eye is illuminated with a blue light.

Lid Eversion. Look at the inner surface of the upper lid while illuminating it with a flashlight. Figure 16-4 shows how to evert an upper lid. Be certain to have the flashlight ready before everting the lid in order to cause the patient only minimal discomfort. There are few things more embarrassing than everting an upper lid, particularly in a noncooperative patient, and then having to let it go because there is not enough light to see the surface detail of the lid.

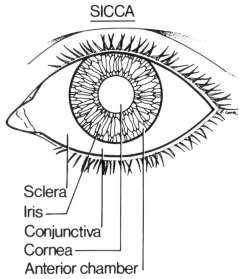

Figure 16-1. Drawing showing five anatomic areas, each of which when affected can produce a red eye. The word SICCA should remind you of sclera, iris, cornea, conjunctiva, and anterior chamber. (Artist: Laurel Cook.)

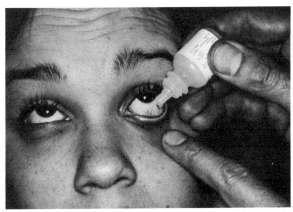

Figure 16-2. To place an eyedrop in the eye, have the patient look up, pull the lower lid down, making a pocket, and place the drop in the pocket.

Lid Evaluation. A quick review of lid structure and function is in order. The lid covers the eye during a blink to keep the cornea moist and clean. The blink must be very rapid so that it does not block vision for any significant amount of time. Therefore, the lid must have a very quick-acting muscle, covered by a thin skin. The skin must be very thin in order to cover the muscle without weighing it down during the blink.

The meibomian glands run along the posterior edges of the lids. These sebaceous-type glands continually secrete tiny amounts of an oily

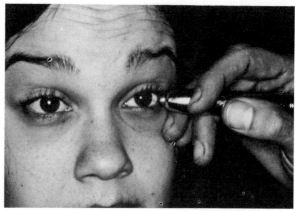

Figure 16-3. Flashlight held at the side of the eye will bring out diseased areas as gray spots on the cornea.

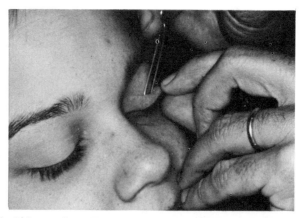

Figure 16-4. Lid eversion. To evert the upper lid (1) have the patient in a comfortable position, (2) have the patient look down, (3) place a clip or cotton-tip applicator along the lid crease, (4) grab the lashes, (5) pull the lashes out and up.

substance onto the margins of the lid. With each blink the oil is layered over the tears. This layer of oil conserves the body's tears by preventing evaporation. An infection or abscess of a meibomian gland is known as a *chalazion.*

The lashes help screen out glare from above and extraneous light reflected from the cheek below. These lashes are kept supple by the meibomian secretion and secretion of the *auxiliary gland* located next to the roots of the lashes. Infection of these auxiliary glands produces a stye.

Conjunctival Redness. A red eye is usually not uniformly red. The redness may be in only one spot (pterygium, episcleritis, or subconjunctival hemorrhage); it may circle the cornea (iritis or central corneal ulcer);

it may appear near one sector of the cornea (peripheral corneal ulcer or abrasion); or the redness may appear primarily on the conjunctival surface of the lid and extend only onto the periphery of the bulbar conjunctiva (conjunctivitis). On occasion, the redness covers the entire white of the eye and is of little value in differential diagnosis.

Pupil. In most cases of acute angle-closure glaucoma, the pupil of the affected eye is larger than that of the fellow eye. The pupil of the affected eye may be smaller than that of the normal eye in cases of corneal abrasion, corneal ulcer, or iritis. In such cases the iris reacts to nearby injury by constricting. The pupil is not affected in conjunctival or episcleral problems.

Finger Pressure. If the diagnosis of acute glaucoma becomes a strong possibility as the clues fall into place, a measurement of intraocular pressure becomes important. In this situation, however, a precise reading of intraocular pressure is not vital. All that is necessary is to know whether the affected eye is much harder than the normal eye. To do this, first gently press through the lid on your own eye to get an idea of normal intraocular pressure. Then gently press on the patient's normal eye (Fig. 16-5). Now compare its resistance to that of the red eye. Is the red eye much firmer than the normal eye? A rock-hard eye suggests glaucoma. On the other hand, a mushy, soft eye suggests a perforating injury through which the fluid contents of the eye have leaked.

Eye Tray

Before we evaluate the eye conditions commonly seen in a generalist's office, let us list the diagnostic equipment needed for a proper eye evaluation. Every emergency room or generalist's office should have an eye tray with the following diagnostic and therapeutic items:

1. Snellen chart

2. Flashlight

3. Fluorescein paper

4. Blue light

5. Dilating medication
   a. Mydriacyl, 1.0%
   b. Scopolamine, 0.3%
   c. Homatropine, 5%
   d. Cyclopentolate, 1%

6. Pilocarpine drops, 4%

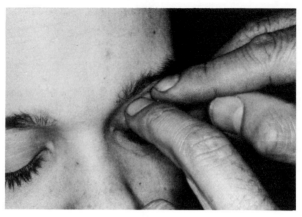

Figure 16-5. Method of palpating the eye through the lid to estimate the intraocular tension.

7. Eye pads

8. Tape

9. Suction cup for contact lens removal

10. Tonometer

11. Cotton-tipped applicators

12. Squeeze bottle of sterile irrigating solution

13. Contact lens wetting solution

14. Roll of pH paper

15. Hand magnet (for metallic corneal foreign bodies)

16. Local anesthetic (0.5% Ophthaine)

17. Disposable, sterile 1-cc or 5-cc syringe with needle (handy, sterile instrument to pick out corneal foreign bodies)

18. Antibiotic eye ointment (any of the following: erythromycin, sulfa, Neosporin®, Chloromycetin®)

19. Magnifying glass

20. Paper clips (to evert or double evert upper lid)

21. Saran Wrap (to cover eyes with badly burned lids).

Problems

The most common problems in an ophthalmology emergency ward are listed in Table 16-1. Many practitioners and internists are uncomfortable treating these ocular emergencies. In this section, the major ocular injuries are discussed and the diagnostic and therapeutic steps that can and should be taken by the family practitioner or emergency room physician are described. The reader should attempt to diagnose the condition presented based on the illustration, the history, and the findings, all of which precede diagnosis, treatment, and discussion. A list of all of the conditions, together with key findings and treatments, appears at the end of this chapter (Table 16-3). Table 16-2 summarizes the diagnoses of acute red eye according to examination results.

Table 16-1. Problems Commonly Encountered in an Ophthalmology Emergency Ward[a]

Condition	Incidence (%)
Corneal foreign body	20
Chalazion	18
Corneal abrasion	12
Conjunctivitis	8
Corneal ulcer	7
Stye	4
Anterior uveitis (iritis)	3
Periorbital cellulitis	2
Subconjunctival hemorrhage	1
Dacryocystitis	< 1
Acute glaucoma	< 1
Chemical splash injury	< 1
Episcleritis	< 1
Other injuries and routine ocular problems	± 20

[a]Reprinted with permission from Price M, Phillips CI: A general practitioner in an ophthalmology accident and emergency department. Br J Med 2:509, 1976.

Table 16–2. Diagnoses of Acute Red Eye According to Examination Results

Test or Question	Response	Diagnosis	Confirmatory Findings
Pain	No	Subconjunctival hemorrhage	Localized dense red lesion with feathery border
	Yes	Others	
Eyes stick together in morning	Yes	Conjunctivitis	Diffuse redness tapering off at limbus
	No	Others	
Visual acuity	Normal	Subconjunctival hemorrhage	
		Conjunctivitis	
		Episcleritis	Local patch of dilated vessels
	Decreased	Corneal disease	
		Iritis	
		Acute glaucoma	
Topical anesthetic relieves pain dramatically	Yes	Corneal disease	Takes fluorescein stain; very photophobic; circumlimbal flush
	No	Acute glaucoma	Tonometry reveals high pressure; ophthalmoscope reveals pulsating retinal artery; steamy cornea

	Tender and firm	Acute glaucoma	(As above)
Pupil size	Small	Iritis	(As above)
	Large	Acute glaucoma	(As above)
Nausea	No	Iritis	(As above)
	Yes	Acute glaucoma	(As above)

Table 16–3. Summary of Common Eye Conditions

Common Condition	Key Findings	Treatment
Conjunctivitis	Eyes stick together, peripheral redness	Antibiotic gtt i q.i.d.
Subconjunctival hemorrhage	Patch of red, feathered edge, no discomfort	Reassurance
Pterygium	Patch of red lines drawn to cornea	0.12% Phenylephrine gtt; refer
Alkali keratoconjunctivitis	History, diffuse redness, decreased vision	Irrigate to pH 7; refer
Penetrating eye injury	History, eye mushy soft	Patch lightly; refer
Anterior uveitis	Photophobia, perilimbal flush, tender to touch	Mydriatics, topical steroids; refer
Acute angle-closure glaucoma	Dull eye pain, nausea, blurred vision, diffuse redness, firm to finger palpation	Refer; pilocarpine, acetazolamide
Episcleritis	Patch of redness, tender	Local steroids; refer
Corneal foreign-body abrasion	History, severe pain relieved by local anesthetic, can see foreign body	Local anesthetic; try to irrigate away; refer
Herpes simplex corneal ulcer	Fluorescein staining dendrite, circumlimbal flush	Local ARA A or IDU

anesthetic

Contact-lens overwear syndrome	Eye pain relieved by local anesthetic, photophobia, history	Remove lenses; antibiotic gtt, sunglasses
Hyphema	History of trauma, blood in anterior chamber, eye pain	Refer; admit to hospital
Hypopyon	As in anterior uveitis, plus pus in anterior chamber	As in anterior uveitis
Ecchymosis (orbital blowout fracture)	Black and blue, lid swelling	Orbital x-ray; check visual acuity; refer if blowout fracture present
Stye	Swollen lid, pointing yellow lesion	Warm compresses q.i.d.
Periorbital cellulitis	Periorbital redness and swelling	Systemic antibiotics, warm compresses
Chalazion	Swollen lid, palpable lump in swollen lid	Warm compresses q.i.d.; refer for incision and drainage if it does not resolve
Dacryocystitis	Local swelling over lacrimal sac, tearing, lids stick together	Systemic antibiotics, warm compresses
Basal-cell carcinoma of lid	Nonhealing lid lesion	Refer for excision
Entropion	Lashes turned in, chronic irritation, chronic tearing	Refer for surgery
Ectropion	Lower-lid droop, tearing	Refer for surgery

Problem 1

History and Examination. The patient's left eye has been irritated and red for several days, and the lids of the left eye stick together upon arising (Fig. 16-6). The results of the examination follow:

Vision	Normal.
Conjunctiva	Redness of peripheral bulbar conjunctiva.
Lids	Some dried exudate on lids.
Cornea	Clear.
Pupils	Symmetric.
Local anesthesia	Makes eye feel better.
Finger tension	Symmetric.

Diagnosis. Conjunctivitis.

Treatment. Antibiotic eyedrops (Neosporin or sulfonamide) are administered to the involved eye 4 times a day for 3–7 days. If the condition does not improve, refer the patient to an ophthalmologist.

Discussion. Inflammation of the conjunctiva may be caused by a host of agents—allergens, physical trauma (fists, dirt, missiles), infective agents, or chemical splashes.

Allergic conjunctivitis usually produces a watery discharge often associated with itching. Local vasoconstrictor agents are helpful. Mild

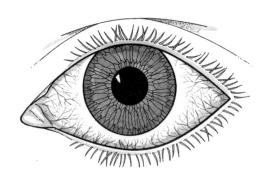

Figure 16-6. Conjunctivitis. (Artists: David Lobel and Laurel Cook.)

physical trauma produces a watery discharge and mild irritation. If severe, physical trauma is associated with secondary infection and thick discharge.

Bacterial conjunctivitis is associated with a thick discharge. The lids stick together upon arising, and there is burning or irritation of the eyes. The administration of a local broad-spectrum antibiotic eyedrop for a few days is the proper treatment.

Viral conjunctivitis is usually associated with a local viral skin rash or upper respiratory infection. It responds symptomatically to local vasoconstrictor drops.

Chemical splashes will be covered later in this section.

Problem 2

History and Examination. The patient arose this morning and noticed a frightening red spot in the white of the eye. The patient reports no pain (Fig. 16-7), but does note vague discomfort. The results of the examination follow:

Vision	Normal.
Lids	Normal.
Conjunctiva	Isolated red area with feathery edge.
Cornea	Clear.
Pupils	Symmetric.
Local anesthesia	Not applicable.
Finger tension	Symmetric.

Diagnosis. Subconjunctival hemorrhage.

Treatment. Ask whether patient has blood-clotting problems. Warm compresses applied to the affected eye 3 times a day for a week will often speed absorption of blood. The condition will take one to three weeks to resolve.

Discussion. Although the condition is usually spontaneous, benign, and unrelated to a systemic problem, it may also be seen with facial and eye trauma, with chest compression, or during labor when the prospective mother bears down. In cases of *eye trauma,* the hemorrhage may overlie a scleral perforation. In such cases an ophthalmologist should be consulted. In rare instances this condition is associated with blood dyscrasia.

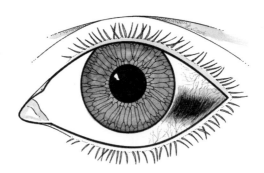

Figure 16-7. Subconjunctival hemorrhage. (Artists: David Lobel and Laurel Cook.)

Problem 3

History and Examination. A red area in corner of the eye has been present for a few years, and recently has begun to feel irritated (Fig. 16-8). The results of the examination follow:

Vision	Normal.
Lids	Normal.
Conjunctiva	Nasal triangular, reddened area on conjunctiva, encroaching on cornea.
Cornea	Leading edge of lesion is gray; under slit lamp, small spots of the cornea next to the lesion take up fluorescein stain.
Pupils	Symmetric.
Local anesthesia	Relieves irritation.
Finger tension	Symmetric.

Diagnosis. Pterygium.

Treatment. Local vasoconstrictor drops (0.12% phenylephrine) 3 times a day often shrink the lesion and decrease the irritation. If such treatment fails, refer the patient to an ophthalmologist for surgical removal of lesion. The ophthalmologist usually will excise the lesion and then arrange for local beta irradiation, which decreases the rate of recurrence of the condition.

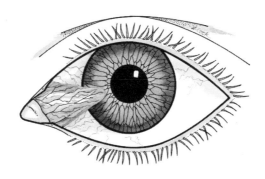

Figure 16-8. Pterygium. (Artists: David Lobel and Laurel Cook.)

Discussion. A *pinguecula* is a yellowish nodule on the sclera, most commonly found on the nasal side of the cornea; the nodule rarely grows and needs no treatment.

A *pterygium* is a pinguecula that has grown, vascularized, and encroached upon the cornea, usually from the nasal side. This phenomenon is common in those who have a history of long exposure to strong sunlight (as in a hot climate). Treatment is indicated when irritation is chronic or when it interferes with vision.

Problem 4

History and Examination. While the patient was mixing plaster, some of it splashed into his eye. The eye is now painful and vision is decreased (Fig. 16-9). The results of the examination follow:

Vision	Decreased in affected eye.
Lids	Some dried pieces of plaster stuck to skin; upon eversion of lid, pieces of plaster stuck to inner lid surface.
Conjunctiva	Uniformly red.
Cornea	Surface epithelium removed in some places; these take up fluorescein dye. Cornea appears hazy.
Pupils	Smaller in affected eye.
Local anesthesia	Makes eye feel much better.
Finger tension	Symmetric.

Diagnosis. Alkali keratoconjunctivitis.

Treatment. Irrigate eye and under lids with sterile solution. Keep checking pH during irrigation by touching pH paper to inner surface of upper lid until neutral pH (7) is achieved.

Dilate pupil with 0.3% scopolamine or 2% homatropine to reduce pain caused by iris spasm.

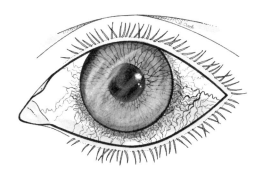

Figure 16-9. Chemical keratoconjunctivitis. (Artists: David Lobel and Laurel Cook.)

Administer antibiotic drops and patch the patient's eye. The patient should take aspirin or another systemic analgesic.

If the patient is not better by the next day, refer him to an ophthalmologist (who may fit patient with soft contact lenses or use local steroids).

Discussion. An alkali burn is much more serious than an acid burn because of its greater tendency to penetrate the depths of the cornea and the interior of the eye. Mild cases usually heal within a week. In severe cases, chronic irritation may last from months to years. If significant corneal opacity develops, the patient ultimately requires a corneal transplant. The prognosis for a clear transplant is, however, poor.

During the early phases of treatment, the corneal epithelium regenerates poorly, and so the lid continually rubs against a raw corneal surface. The ophthalmologist often uses a soft contact lens as a transparent bandage to prevent this rubbing and to allow epithelial healing.

Problem 5

History and Examination. The patient's eye was poked by a pencil. The eye is now painful and vision is poor (Fig. 16-10). The results of the examination follow:

Vision	Decreased in involved eye.
Lids	Normal.
Conjunctiva	Redness, mostly in area of injury; black area next to limbus.
Cornea	Slightly wrinkled.
Pupil	Irregular in shape.
Local anesthesia	Some decrease in the pain.
Finger tension	Involved eye is mushy soft.

Diagnosis. Penetrating eye injury.

Treatment. Administer systemic analgesics and a tetanus-toxoid booster, and apply a sterile bandage on the closed eye.

Refer the patient to an ophthalmologist, who will (1) x-ray eye or use a diagnostic ultrasound unit to determine if foreign material is still present in eye, and (2) surgically repair laceration.

Discussion. In about half of the cases, a penetrating wound is repaired and vision regained, but through-and-through wounds have a poor prognosis. Depending on the site and the extent of the injury, the patient may develop iritis, cataract, glaucoma, retinal detachment, vitreous hemorrhage, or corneal scarring. When a number of these complications arise, and when it appears that the eye will never see properly and may be chronically painful, enucleation is often recommended.

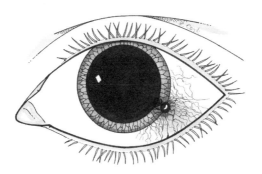

Figure 16-10. Penetrating eye injury. (Artists: David Lobel and Laurel Cook.)

Problem 6

History and Examination. The patient experiences ocular pain associated with blurred vision and sensitivity to light (Fig. 16-11). The results of the examination follow:

Vision	Decreased in affected eye.
Lids	Normal.
Conjunctiva	Mildly red, with increase in redness in circumlimbal area.
Cornea	Grossly clear under slit-lamp observation, many gray spots (called keratic precipitates or "KPs") can be seen on back surface of cornea.
Pupils	Smaller in affected eye; slit-lamp examination reveals fine cells floating in anterior chamber.
Local anesthesia	Irritation only slightly improved.
Finger tension	Affected eye tender to the touch; both eyes appear to have the same tension.

Diagnosis. Anterior uveitis.

Treatment. Check for presence of associated systemic diseases (sarcoidosis, rheumatoid arthritis, tuberculosis, Reiter's syndrome), and dilate the pupil.

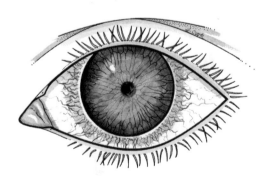

Figure 16-11. Anterior uveitis. (Artists: David Lobel and Laurel Cook.)

Refer the patient to an ophthalmologist, who will (1) monitor intraocular pressure (glaucoma is the most frequent complication and may be due to posterior or anterior synechiae formation or, during the acute period, may be due to inflammatory cells impeding aqueous outflow); (2) start local corticosteroid eyedrops; and (3) thoroughly examine eye for presence of posterior uveitis.

Discussion. Anterior uveitis (often called iritis) is a potentially dangerous disease if not treated immediately, leading to glaucoma and/or cataract. Referral to an ophthalmologist is important. Anterior uveitis usually presents as a red, painful eye. The important exception is children who develop anterior uveitis in association with juvenile rheumatoid arthritis. These children have uninflamed eyes and a minimum of anterior uveitis. For full discussion of this condition refer to Chapter 12.

Problem 7

History and Examination. The patient experiences sudden onset of eye pain and blurring of vision associated with nausea and vomiting (Fig. 16-12). The results of the examination follow:

Vision	Decreased in affected eye.
Lids	Normal.
Conjunctiva	Diffusely red right up to circumlimbal region.
Cornea	Slightly hazy compared to normal eye.
Pupils	Enlarged and nonreactive to light on affected side.
Local anesthesia	No effect.
Finger tension	Involved eye feels rock-hard compared to normal eye.

Diagnosis. Acute angle-closure glaucoma.

Treatment. Apply one drop of 4% pilocarpine ophthalmic preparation in involved eye every 20 minutes.

Immediately administer acetazolamide 250 mg by mouth.

Refer the patient to an ophthalmologist, who probably will (1) reduce the pressure medically with continued use of pilocarpine; (2) administer

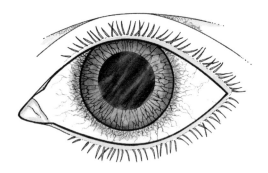

Figure 16-12. Acute angle-closure glaucoma. (Artists: David Lobel and Laurel Cook.)

50% glycerine preparation orally or use intravenous hyperosmotic agent (mannitol, urea); and (3) when intraocular pressure is normal, perform surgical procedure known as peripheral iridectomy, usually under local anesthesia.

Discussion. It should be noted that an acute attack of angle-closure glaucoma may blind the patient if left untreated. Although the immediate treatment is medical, a cure can ultimately be effected only with surgical intervention. For full discussion refer to Chapter 9.

Problem 8

History and Examination. One of the patient's eyes has been tender and irritated for several days (Fig. 16-13). The results of the examination follow:

Vision	Normal in both eyes.
Lids	Normal.
Conjunctiva	Local raised area of redness, slit-lamp examination reveals that the dilated vessels are primarily in the deep episcleral tissue, and these deeper vessels look violet as opposed to the red of the superficial conjunctival vessels.
Cornea	Clear in both eyes.
Pupils	Symmetric.
Local anesthesia	Relieves most of the irritation.
Finger tension	Symmetric in the two eyes, but involved eye is tender to the touch.

Diagnosis. Episcleritis.

Treatment. Check for presence of associated systemic diseases, such as rheumatoid arthritis or other collagen diseases. Then apply corticosteroid eyedrops 3 times daily.

Since this is a difficult diagnosis to make, do not hesitate to obtain the opinion of an ophthalmologist.

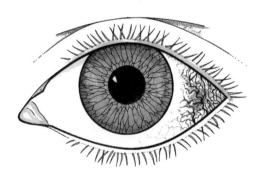

Figure 16-13. Episcleritis. (Artists: David Lobel and Laurel Cook.)

Discussion. Episcleritis is a circumscribed nodular inflammation of the episcleral tissue (thin layer between conjunctiva and sclera) causing discomfort rather than pain. The inflamed episcleral vessels (more purple than the conjunctival vessels) appear within the interpalpebral fissure. A single attack, untreated, lasts for two months. The condition can be associated with systemic collagen vascular disease, skin disease (e.g., psoriasis), allergic conditions, and gout.[1]

Scleritis is an inflammation of the collagen of the sclera, associated with severe pain, diminished vision (often), and ultimately scleral thinning, which may proceed to perforation of the globe. The duration of an attack may range from months to years. The lesion is usually covered by the lid. Scleritis is usually associated with the collagen vascular diseases.[2] For example, there is a syndrome consisting of scleritis, rheumatoid nodules, arteritis, and pleurisy.[3] Treatment consists of prolonged use of systemic antiinflammatory agents (steroids, oxyphenbutazone, aspirin).

Problem 9

History and Examination. The patient reports feeling intense pain in one eye after striking piece of metal with a hammer (Fig. 16-14). The results of the examination follow:

Vision	Slightly decreased in involved eye.
Lids	Normal.
Conjunctiva	Reddened, with more intense area of redness near cornea in area of foreign body.
Cornea	Dark speck embedded in cornea; when fluorescein dye is applied, area around foreign body takes up dye.
Pupil	Smaller in affected eye.
Local anesthesia	Relieves foreign body sensation.
Finger tension	Symmetric in the two eyes.

Diagnosis. Corneal foreign body.

Treatment. Attempt to remove foreign body by irrigating cornea with stream from irrigation bottle. If history suggests that the foreign body is metal, hold magnet close to eye in attempt to draw off foreign body. If these maneuvers fail, attempt to remove foreign body with sterile needle under magnification. Do not attempt this maneuver unless you have been specially trained.

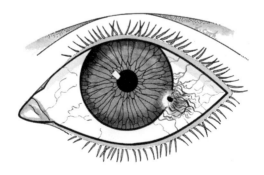

Figure 16-14. Corneal limbal foreign body. (Artists: David Lobel and Laurel Cook.)

After foreign body is removed, treat the case as a corneal abrasion. Dilate the pupil with a drop of 0.3% scopolamine or 2% homatropine to break pupillary spasm; place antibiotic solution or antibiotic ointment in eye; patch the eye only if the patient feels more comfortable with the patch in place; and inspect the wound daily until healed.

If you are unable to remove foreign body, refer the patient to an ophthalmologist.

Discussion. If the foreign body is iron, a brown coloration (rust or char from hot metal) may appear at the base of the lesion. The application of antibiotic ointment occasionally loosens this rust deposit and the foreign body may spontaneously fall out in a day or two. If the brown deposit remains, reepithelialization is inhibited, and the ophthalmologist will have to scrape away the brown bed so that proper healing can take place.

Problem 10

History and Examination. The patient has experienced moderate pain, redness, and decreased vision in one eye for the past few days. He had a similar condition about a year ago, and was told that it was an ulcer (Fig. 16-15). The results of the examination follow:

Vision	Decreased in involved eye.
Lids	Normal.
Conjunctiva	Diffusely red, with circumlimbal flush.
Cornea	Fine gray area seen with flashlight; after the application of fluorescein, branched pattern of fluorescein seen on corneal surface.
Pupils	Smaller on affected side.
Local anesthesia	Relieves most of the irritation.
Finger tension	Symmetric in the two eyes.

Diagnosis. Herpes simplex corneal ulcer.

Treatment. Apply iododeoxyuridine (IDU) ointment or ARA-A eye ointment or drops to the affected eye every 2 hours.

Dilate pupil with 0.3% scopolamine drops.

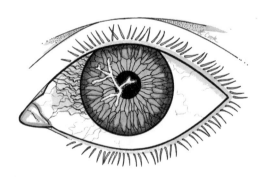

Figure 16-15. Herpes simplex corneal ulcer. (Artists: David Lobel and Laurel Cook.)

If there is no response in 2–3 days, refer to ophthalmologist. The ophthalmologist may either continue medication or scrape off surface cells of cornea.

Discussion. Unhappily, this disease sometimes recurs, and subsequent episodes may involve the corneal stroma. If this occurs, the disease becomes long-term and produces chronic irritation, decreased vision, and photophobia. Repeated attacks may lead to corneal scarring, which may ultimately necessitate a corneal transplant.

Problem 11

History and Examination. Pain, redness, and blurred vision in one eye for past few days (Fig. 16-16). The results of the examination follow:

Vision	Decreased in involved eye.
Conjunctiva	Diffusely red with increase in redness in perilimbal region.
Cornea	Irregular gray-white area in cornea; these areas take up fluorescein stain.
Pupils	Smaller on affected side.
Local anesthesia	Relieves pain.
Finger tension	Symmetric.

Diagnosis. Bacterial or fungal ulcer.

Treatment. This patient should be referred to an ophthalmologist immediately. The ophthalmologist will scrape the ulcerated area and send a specimen for smear, as well as for culture and sensitivity studies, to determine what microorganism is responsible for the infection. He or she will also administer an appropriate antibiotic (drops, ointment, or subconjunctival injection).

Discussion. A number of situations seem to predispose the cornea to bacterial or fungal ulceration. Among them are neglected foreign-body injuries to the cornea, comatose patients whose lid-closure is not complete, chronic alcoholics who neglect themselves, and, finally, careless contact-lens wearers who overwear their lenses or do not clean them properly. For specifics on antibiotic therapy, refer to Chapter 14.

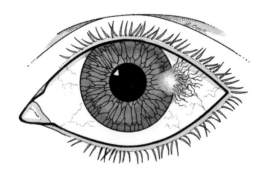

Figure 16-16. Bacterial corneal ulcer. (Artists: David Lobel and Laurel Cook.)

Problem 12

History and Examination. Acid was splashed into the eye of the patient and the eye became red and painful. The patient reports blurred vision (Fig. 16-17). The results of the examination follow:

Vision	Decreased in involved eye.
Lids	Some evidence of acid burn (on skin of face also).
Conjunctiva	Diffusely red.
Cornea	Gray in appearance.
Pupil	Smaller in involved eye.
Local anesthesia	Relieves pain.
Finger tension	Symmetric.

Diagnosis. Chemical corneal burn.

Treatment. Irrigate eye and under lids copiously. Continue irrigation until pH paper (applied to undersurface of lid) is neutral.

Dilate the pupil with a single administration of 0.3% scopolamine eyedrops.

Apply antibiotic eyedrop.

Administer systemic analgesic.

Refer to ophthalmologist, who will probably use local corticosteroids, apply a continuous-wear soft contact lens that fosters reepithelialization of the cornea, and ultimately perform a corneal transplant if the cornea does not clear.

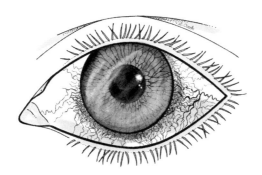

Figure 16-17. Acid burn of the cornea. (Artists: David Lobel and Laurel Cook.)

Discussion. Mild acid burns usually heal within a week. Severe acid burns are not as serious as alkali burns because the acid tends to denature and coagulate corneal-surface proteins; the coagulum forms a barrier to further damage. In these patients, chronic irritation is not a problem. If the damage is great enough, dense corneal scarring may result and, if vision is severely impaired, corneal transplantation may be necessary. Such patients have a fairly good prognosis for a successful corneal transplantation.

Problem 13

History and Examination. A young woman enters the emergency room covering both eyes. She reports that her eyes hurt and that bright light annoys her. She also says that she overwore her contact lenses last night and, after a few hours of sleep, was aroused by severe pain in both eyes (Fig. 16-18). The results of the examination follow:

Vision	Will not open eyes until anesthetic is placed in each eye. She then reports a decrease in vision in each eye.
Lids	Normal.
Conjunctiva	Diffusely red.
Cornea	Grossly clear, but under slit-lamp observation with fluorescein-dye administration many small fluorescein-staining spots dot the surface of each cornea.
Pupils	Both somewhat small.
Local anesthesia	Relieves pain.
Finger tension	Symmetric.

Diagnosis. Contact lens overwear syndrome.

Treatment. Administer systemic analgesics (aspirin, etc.).

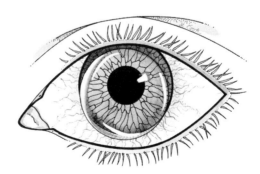

Figure 16-18. Contact-lens overwear syndrome. (Artists: David Lobel and Laurel Cook.)

Dilate pupils with short-acting mydriatic such as 1% cyclopentolate.

Suggest using sunglasses until symptoms abate (the corneal surface will heal in 1–2 days).

Stop use of contact lenses until all symptoms are gone.

Refer to eye doctor to have fit of the contact lenses checked.

Discussion. In almost all of these cases, early therapy prevents complications and the patient is back to wearing contact lenses in less than a week.

Problem 14

History and Examination. The patient was struck in the eye with tennis ball, and now reports pain and blurred vision in that eye (Fig. 16-19). The results of the examination follow:

Vision	Decreased in involved eye.
Lids	May be slightly swollen.
Conjunctiva	Diffusely red.
Cornea	Probably has surface abrasion; under slit-lamp examination, central area takes up fluorescein dye.
Pupil	Smaller on side of injury—*note level of blood in anterior chamber.*
Local anesthesia	Relieves much of the irritation.
Finger tension	Affected eye may feel slightly harder than fellow eye.

Diagnosis. Hyphema.

Treatment. Five days of bed-rest (hospitalize if the patient is a child or lives alone).

Consult with, and refer the patient to, an ophthalmologist. The condition is potentially very serious and often leads to acute glaucoma. In the event of a rehemorrhage, the ophthalmologist may be forced to perform an operation in which he aspirates the blood from the eye.

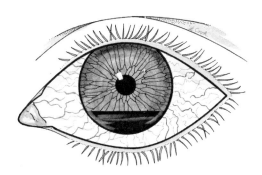

Figure 16-19. Hyphema. (Artists: David Lobel and Laurel Cook.)

Discussion. This patient's greatest problem is to avoid a second hemorrhage, which is usually much worse than the original. The patient is patched bilaterally for 5 days to decrease his interest in his surroundings and to encourage rest. Rehemorrhage is often followed by acute glaucoma; this is first treated medically (acetazolamide or such hyperosomotic agents as mannitol or urea). The blood is evacuated surgically if medical treatment fails.

Problem 15

History and Examination. The patient's eye has been irritated and red for the past few days, with a decrease in vision (Fig. 16-20). The results of the examination follow:

Vision	Decreased in involved eye.
Lids	Normal.
Conjunctiva	Redness primarily perilimbal.
Cornea	Often clear.
Pupil	Smaller on affected side; pus in anterior chamber.
Local anesthesia	Little effect on irritation.
Finger tension	Symmetric.

Diagnosis. Hypopyon.

Treatment. This patient has a severe form of iritis and should be referred to an ophthalmologist. The ophthalmologist will probably treat with corticosteroid eyedrops, dilate the pupil with scopolamine or atropine drops, monitor the intraocular pressure, and medically treat any episode of glaucoma.

Discussion. Except for cases of associated endophthalmitis or penetrating ocular trauma, the pus in the anterior chamber is almost always sterile in anterior uveitis. The fact that a very small group of patients develops hypopyon after cataract surgery or after soft-contact-lens overwear suggests an exaggerated intraocular inflammatory response in these patients, in whom the exudation from the uvea is increased dramatically.

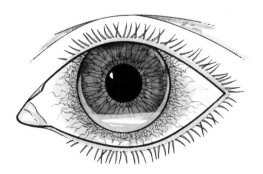

Figure 16-20. Hypopyon. (Artists: David Lobel and Laurel Cook.)

Problem 16

History and Examination. A young man was struck in one eye with a fist, and now reports a swollen lid (Fig. 16-21). The results of the examination follow:

Vision	Swollen lid may preclude accurate examination of vision; if visual acuity can be recorded, it is usually normal.
Lids	Swollen and ecchymotic due to ruptured subcutaneous blood vessels, may have decreased skin sensation under lower lid.
Conjunctiva	Often mildly red.
Cornea	Clear.
Pupil	Occasionally dilated and unreactive to light, small amounts of blood may sometimes be seen in the anterior chamber under slit-lamp examination (hyphema).
Local anesthesia	Little effect on feeling of discomfort.
Finger tension	Cannot feel eyeball through the swollen lid, but sometimes the examiner feels a crackling crepitus within the lid; this suggests the presence of air, which has probably invaded the tissue from a fracture of the wall of the ethmoid sinus.

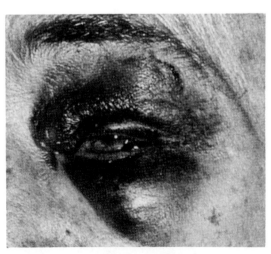

Figure 16-21. Ecchymosis (orbital blowout fracture).

| Eye movement | With swollen eyelid raised, patient often reports double vision. |

Diagnosis. Ecchymosis.

Treatment. A black eye is a potentially serious problem. To determine its severity, obtain x-ray of orbits. A fracture of the floor of the orbit (blowout fracture) necessitates an ophthalmologic evaluation. (This fracture often causes inferior rectus muscle entrapment.)

The presence of double vision is a signal for referral to an ophthalmologist. Persistent diplopia may necessitate surgical intervention. Decreased vision in the traumatized eye also demands referral.

If the eye and orbit are normal, cold compresses should relieve the swelling.

Once all swelling subsides, a thorough ocular examination is necessary to rule out subtle retinal contusions or tears, as well as other damage that might lead to glaucoma.

Discussion. Persistent, annoying diplopia with the straight-ahead gaze and cosmetically distorting endophthalmos are the two indications for surgical correction of a blowout fracture. Surgical correction involves a significant risk to the optic nerve and should not be undertaken lightly.

From a philosophical point of view, one may look at severe ecchymosis as nature's way of administering a pressure dressing to keep the eyes closed and moist for a few days. Such a device would be helpful in cases of head trauma associated with unconsciousness.

Problem 17

History and Examination. The patient has painful swelling on the margin of his lid (Fig. 16-22). The results of the examination follow:

Vision	Normal.
Lid	Local swelling, which appears to be coming to a yellow head, between the lashes of the lid.
Conjunctiva	Mildly pink.
Cornea	Clear.
Pupils	Symmetric.
Local anesthesia	Does not relieve irritation substantially.
Finger tension	Lid tender, symmetric tension.

Diagnosis. Stye.

Treatment. Apply warm compresses, 10 minutes per application, 4 times per day, until lesion erupts and drains. The use of antibiotic drops or ointment is of little value.

Discussion. The lashes help screen out glare light from above and extraneous light reflected from the cheek below. These lashes are kept supple by the meibomian secretion and secretion from the auxiliary gland located right next to the roots of the lashes. Infection of these auxiliary glands produces a stye. A recurrent stye suggests that the patient continually introduces high levels of microorganisms into his eye, probably by rubbing his eyes. Such a chain of events is often seen in patients who touch or pick the nose and then rub the eyes.

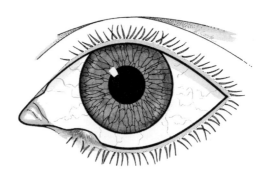

Figure 16-22. Stye. (Artists: David Lobel and Laurel Cook.)

Problem 18

History and Examination. The patient reports a sudden onset of swelling that seems to have spread all around the right eye. He cannot recall injury to face or being bitten by an insect (Fig. 16-23). The results of the examination follow:

Vision	Normal.
Lid	Red swelling of lid and periorbital area; occasionally the examiner finds an infected hair follicle, which may have been the initial site of infection.
Conjunctiva	Mildly red.
Cornea	Clear.
Pupils	Symmetric.
Local anesthesia	Not applicable.
Finger tension	Tender, swollen lid, cannot easily feel eyeball beneath swelling.

Diagnosis. Periorbital cellulitis.

Treatment. If there is a draining site on the skin, collect a specimen and order culture and susceptibility tests.

Immediately start systemic administration of a potent antibiotic.

Apply warm compresses, 10 minutes at a time, 4 times a day.

Follow the patient daily. If there is no improvement in 1–2 days, hospitalize the patient and start intravenous antibiotics.

Discussion. Orbital cellulitis often results from a secondarily infected wound or from a preexisting furuncle; in such cases, obtain exudate for cultures and order susceptibility tests to help in choosing proper antibiotic treatment. Since the most common organism is *Staphylococcus aureus,* one often starts empirical treatment with one of the penicillins. The condition is serious, because some of the subcutaneous veins around the orbit drain directly into the brain's venous system. The infection, if unchecked, can lead directly to the brain.

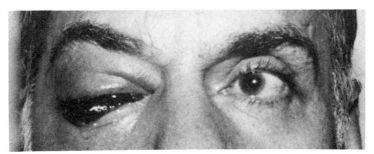

Figure 16-23. Periorbital cellulitis. (Courtesy of Gary Griffiths.)

The differential diagnosis of nonhemorrhagic periorbital swelling, particularly if associated with trauma, includes (1) infection, (2) allergy, and (3) cerebrospinal leak. The mechanism of the swelling in each of these conditions is a combination of vasodilation and excess interstitial fluid. In infection, the swollen area appears red because of the large vasodilatory component, and the pain is of a throbbing nature. In allergy, the swelling is mostly due to fluid leaking from partially dilated vessels. Thus, the swelling is more translucent or cystic and may be associated with itching. A cerebrospinal leak also produces a translucent, cystic swelling (which may not be throbbing and painful) that is associated with severe frontal bone trauma.

Finally, it is interesting that the lid can swell more than the skin covering other structures. The lid, of course, moistens and cleans the cornea with each blink, and the blink must be fast enough to keep the vision clear. Therefore, the lid must have a very quick-acting muscle covered by skin thin enough to cover the muscle without weighing it down during the blink. Thus, the thin skin offers little resistance to the underlying edema.

Problem 19

History and Examination. The patient has been afflicted with painful swelling of the lid for about a week (Fig. 16-24). The results of the examination follow:

Vision	Slightly blurred in involved eye; lump pushes on the eyeball, inducing small amount of astigmatism.
Lid	Lid eversion reveals discrete red lump.
Conjunctiva	Mildly red.
Cornea	Clear.
Pupils	Symmetric.
Local anesthesia	Little effect on pain.
Finger tension	Mass can be outlined within lid; tension is symmetric.

Diagnosis. Chalazion.

Treatment. Apply warm compresses for 10 minutes 4 times a day.

If the response to the compresses is poor, refer the patient to an ophthalmologist. The ophthalmologist will incise and drain the lesion.

Discussion. A chalazion (from the Greek for "small hailstone") is a chronic inflammatory granuloma that shows giant cells on histologic section.

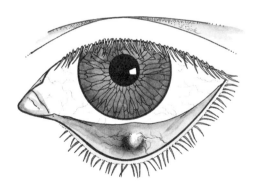

Figure 16-24. Chalazion. (Artists: David Lobel and Laurel Cook.)

This condition is usually the result of obstruction of one of the meibomian glands. Secretions from these glands keep the lashes supple. Continued secretion produces a cystic swelling that becomes secondarily infected (usually with *Staphylococcus aureus*). The wall of the inflamed gland sometimes ruptures, evoking an inflammatory reaction. Reactive lid swelling can become very large in some cases. Interestingly, chalazions rarely produce secondary corneal infection. Some patients who suffer from recurrent chalazions ultimately develop lid-scarring, which can interfere with tear drainage and produce annoying tearing.

Since meibomian secretion is closely related to sebum, one can almost think of a chalazion as a local form of an acne comedo. In both conditions, abnormal keratinization of the follicle or gland wall leads to occlusion and accumulation of secretion, bacteria, and keratinous material. Rupture of the cyst wall spews the oily secretion into the tissues, inducing a giant-cell, foreign-body response.

Problem 20

History and Examination. The patient has suffered from progressive, painful red swelling in the area between the nose and eye for the past few days. The eyes also tear and the lids stick together in the morning (Fig. 16-25). The results of the examination follow:

Vision	Normal.
Lid	Lower lid mildly swollen; area over lacrimal sac tender and swollen.
Conjunctiva	Normal or mildly red.
Cornea	Clear; excess tearing noted.
Pupils	Symmetric.
Local anesthesia	Not applicable.
Finger tension	Symmetric.

Diagnosis. Dacryocystitis.

Treatment. If area is fluctuant, incision and drainage are indicated. If nonfluctuant, apply warm compresses to bring to a head.

Administer a systemic antibiotic.

If the condition does not respond, the patient may require hospitalization and surgical excision of the lacrimal sac.

Discussion. A retrograde secondary bacterial conjunctivitis always accompanies this condition because of the obstruction of tear flow. Since the lesion is deep, treatment consists of systemic antibiotics. The possible sequelae include (1) orbital cellulitis and (2) stenosis of the nasolacrimal system. This latter condition may ultimately necessitate the surgical construction of a new tear passageway between lid and nose.

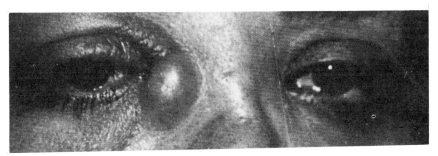

Figure 16-25. Dacryocystitis.

Problem 21

History and Examination. The patient reports an ulcer on the lid that has been present for a few months and that does not heal (Fig. 16-26). The results of the examination follow:

Vision	Normal.
Lid	Elevated skin lesion with ulcerated surface.
Conjunctiva	Normal.
Cornea	Clear.
Pupils	Symmetric.
Local anesthesia	Not applicable.
Finger tension	Symmetric.

Diagnosis. Basal-cell carcinoma.

Treatment. Photograph the lesion and treat with local antibiotic ointment and warm compresses.

If it does not heal in a few weeks, refer the patient to an ophthalmologist. The ophthalmologist will biopsy the lesion. If malignant, he will either excise the lesion—along with a generous disease-free border—or destroy the lesion with x-ray or cryotherapy.

Discussion. Since this lesion rarely metastasizes, the situation is not life-threatening. If the lesion enlarges, however, it does threaten normal ocular function. Specifically, wide excision of a large lesion makes reconstruction difficult. Such a patient is often left with a reconstructed lid which is not normal in appearance, which may not wet the cornea properly, or which may not help drain tears efficiently. Thus, the excision of a large lid lesion should be referred to a plastic ophthalmic surgeon.

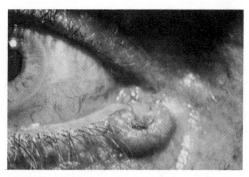

Figure 16-26. Basal-cell carcinoma of the lid. (Reprinted with permission from Fraunfelder FT, Wallace TR, Farris HE, et al: The role of cryosurgery in external ocular and periocular disease. Trans Am Acad Ophthalmol Otolaryngol 83:713–724, 1977.)

Problem 22

History and Examination. An elderly patient has been afflicted with an irritated red eye for the past few months. The patient also reports mild sensitivity to light (Fig. 16-27). The results of the examination follow:

Vision	Normal.
Lids	Lower lid curled inward with lashes rubbing against cornea.
Conjunctiva	Mildly inflamed around lower border of limbus.
Cornea	Clear grossly; under slit-lamp observation, many small areas on lower third of cornea take up the fluorescein stain.
Pupils	Symmetric.
Local anesthesia	Eliminates irritation.
Finger tension	Not applicable.

Diagnosis. Entropion.

Treatment. A chronically abraded cornea is a potentially serious condition; interruption of the epithelial barrier provides a greater possibility of corneal infection. Thus, antibiotic ointment should be administered to the affected eye.

Pluck inturned lashes.

If the condition progresses, the patient should be referred to an ophthalmologist, who probably will reestablish the correct lid position with surgery.

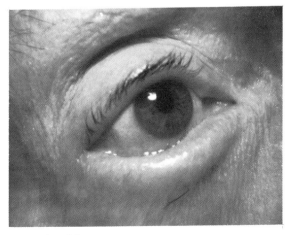

Figure 16-27. Entropion lid.

Discussion. With aging, absorption of orbital fat produces some degree of endophthalmos, reducing the pressure of the globe against the lid. On the other side, the atonia of the lid muscle and relaxation of the lid skin also reduce pressure of the lid against the globe. Eventually, support of the lower tarsus ebbs to the point where the lower tarsus falls forward and the tissue at the superior edge of the lower tarsal plate rotates backward toward the eye. Surgical repair involves tightening the lax tissue.

Problem 23

History and Examination. An elderly patient has had a red, irritated, and unsightly eye for a number of months (Fig. 16-28). The results of the examination follow:

Vision	Normal.
Lid	The lower lid is turned out, reddened, and thickened.
Conjunctiva	The lower part of the eye is reddened.
Cornea	Clear grossly; under slit-lamp observation, many small areas in the lower third of the cornea take up the fluorescein stain.
Pupils	Symmetric.
Local anesthesia	Eliminates irritation.
Finger tension	Not applicable.

Diagnosis. Ectropion.

Treatment. As a first step, antibiotic ointments and artificial tears can be applied to the cornea to keep it moist. Warm compresses may relieve the secondary lid swelling.

If the condition progresses, the patient should be referred to an ophthalmologist, who can reestablish the correct lid position surgically.

Discussion. The lower part of the cornea is kept chronically dry and unmoistened by the everted, drooping lower lid. The epithelial cells dry

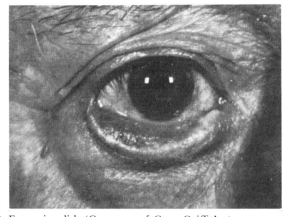

Figure 16-28. Ectropion lid. (Courtesy of Gary Griffiths.)

out and die, leaving the cornea more vulnerable to infection. In the elderly this condition is caused by the inevitable, progressive atonia of lid muscles and by the decreased elasticity of the lid skin and fascia. Early in the course of the lid sag, the nasolacrimal duct may become kinked, and excess tearing may be an early symptom. As the lid sags further, the cornea dries, producing ocular irritation and accompanying tearing.

Summary

We have tried, almost in cookbook fashion, to review the emergency management of 23 commonly encountered eye conditions (see Table 16-3). In such cases, the key principles of management include the following:

1. Maintaining a well-equipped eye tray.

2. Performing a methodic ocular examination in each case.

3. Using a topical anesthetic, with little hesitation, in order to make the patient feel more comfortable and to allow a proper examination.

4. Refraining from placing ointment in the eye of a patient about to be referred to an ophthalmologist. The ointment will interfere with his examination.

5. X-raying every "black eye."

6. Obtaining help when unsure.

References

1. Lyne AJ, Pit Keathley DA: Episcleritis and scleritis. Arch Ophthalmol 80:171, 1968

2. Long RG, Friedmann AI, James DG: Scleritis and temporal arteritis. Postgrad Med J 52:689, 1976

3. Hazleman BL: Ocular manifestations of rheumatic diseases. Practitioner 217:83, 1978

Chapter 17

Eye Myths

Myths are by definition fictitious and eyes are historically a major focus for superstition. The evil eye can be averted if you have salt in your pockets. People who squint are dishonest. The best man in a wedding is a decoy to attract the evil eye away from the groom. Sweeping a black cat's tail across your eyes daily will prevent cataracts. Reliable people look you straight in the eye. If you wear your rubbers in the house, you will go blind.

We could go on indefinitely with myths, superstitions, and old wives' tales, and we could all smile and laugh knowing that they are all unfounded but nonetheless funny. The "quiz" that follows deals with some common misconceptions and truisms, and should take three to five minutes for you to review.

True or False?

1. *Women are more attractive if they wear eye make-up.* The truth (beauty) is in the eye of the beholder, but the corneal abrasion or infection may be in the eye of the beheld. Be aware that these may be complications of wearing eye make-up.

2. *Children will probably outgrow crossed eyes in time.* False. Crossed eyes in children are always a serious condition and require an eye doctor's care. In some cases the eyes only appear to cross; the problem may be related not to muscle weakness but to lid skin partially covering the eye. Only in this instance will time lessen the problem.

3. *Children with measles may go blind if they are exposed to bright light.* False. Measles and photophobia are often related since the measles virus often invades the cornea to produce a keratitis. An irritated cornea is almost always associated with light sensitivity. Thus, the child is more comfortable in a darkened room or wearing dark glasses. Exposure to bright light will cause no permanent damage.

4. *Night vision can be improved if you increase the number of carrots (or amount of vitamin A) in the diet.* False. Most people get enough vitamin A in their diets to supply their eyes adequately. In the rare case of vitamin A deficiency, the improvement will obviously relate to vitamin A intake.

5. *A blue eye should not be used for transplanting into a brown-eyed person.* False. The cornea is the only part of the eye that is ever transplanted. It is clear and does not change the eye color of the recipient.

6. *The incidence of nearsightedness is increasing in modern society.* True. Not too long ago a study was carried out to determine the refractive status of the Eskimos in Point Barrow, Alaska. The study revealed that whereas the older (illiterate) members of the community had excellent distance vision, the youngsters, who were all in school, showed significant nearsightedness.

7. *A cataract is actually a film over the eye which can be peeled off surgically.* False. Cataracts develop in the lens of the eye. Therefore the lens must be removed if the cataract is to be removed.

8. *Excessive radiation, as from sun exposure, can stimulate the formation of cataracts.* This is being studied at the University of Rochester. Evidence gathered so far in studies on animals indicates that this may be true.

9. *Cataracts sometimes grow back after cataract surgery.* False. Once a lens is removed completely, it will not grow back. On occasion some of the lens is not removed at surgery; if this should occur, an "after-cataract" can recur.

10. *Cataracts have to be 'ripe' before surgery can be performed.* False. With today's surgical techniques, cataracts can be removed whenever the patient is significantly bothered by them.

11. *Glare bothers people who have cataracts.* True. Cataracts diffuse light, blurring the images. Bright light tends to exaggerate this effect.

12. *Headaches are usually due to eye strain.* False. The most common cause of headaches is tension. If the headaches persist, a medical examination is indicated. If the headaches are related to significant eye problems (pain, blurring, etc.), an ophthalmologic consultation is in order.

13. *Seeing is an art that can be improved with exercises.* False. Proponents of Dr. William Bates (1900–1930), the most expressive of whom was Aldous Huxley, and the most recent of whom are the health faddists, will argue that this is definitely true. But studies done since the 1950s have been unable to support this argument. Today, the general consensus among ophthalmologists and optometrists is that this is false. Nevertheless, eye exercises can sometimes improve attention.

14. *Children who have a problem learning to read are likely to have an eye-coordination problem and can be helped with special exercises.* False. All controlled studies have proven this to be false (see No. 13). Unfortunately, believing or desperate parents will pay fraudulent or naive educators and others on this premise.

15. *Children should be taught not to hold their books too close while reading since this can harm their eyes.* False. All eyes, and particularly children's, are adaptable. The function of the lens is to focus light, and using accommodation will not harm the eyes. If a child cannot focus on distant objects, however, he or she should be given a vision test.

16. *Reading for prolonged periods in dim light can harm the eyes.* False. See No. 15. It may be difficult or uncomfortable or cause a headache, but it will not harm the eyes.

17. *Older people who may be having trouble seeing should not use their eyes too much since they can wear them out sooner.* False. The eyes cannot wear out with use.

18. *People with weak eyes should rest their eyes often in order to strengthen them.* False. Eyes do not become weak by use and do not become strong by rest.

19. *If children sit too close to the TV set they may damage their eyes.* False. See No. 15. Now that the radiation hazards of color TV sets have been controlled, sitting close is no longer unsafe for any known reason.

20. *Watching TV is bad for the eyes.* False. See No. 16.

21. *Light-adjustable TV receivers are less fatiguing to the eyes than other types.* Sharp contrasts in light and dark mean that more precise accommodation must take place in the lens. This will not harm the lens in any way. There is no reason why light-adjustable televisions might be less fatiguing, if indeed they are.

22. *Wearing glasses that are too strong can damage the eyes.* False. Damage will be caused only to the images viewed. If you do not mind the blurring, then wear the strong glasses; your eyes will not suffer.

23. *Nearsighted people may outgrow their need for glasses, since they will become farsighted as they grow older.* False. Presbyopia comes with age. As the

condition progresses and accommodation is lost, the patient must hold objects farther away in order to see them clearly. This has nothing to do with nearsightedness.

24. *A sign of healthy eyes in old people is their ability to read the newspaper without glasses.* False. It means only that they are nearsighted, either since birth or since the development of a cataract, which may cause an eye to become nearsighted, hence "second sight."

25. *People who wear glasses should be checked every year to see if a lens change is needed.* False. Lenses need to be changed only when the wearer cannot see clearly anymore. Frames need to be changed when the wearer wants to move with the fashions.

26. *Wearing glasses makes you dependent on them.* False. Glasses are not addicting. Seeing clearly, however, is.

27. *Not wearing glasses when you need them makes your eyes worse.* False. Eyes are neither aided nor harmed by glasses—images are. Not wearing needed glasses will distort the images, but will not harm the eyes.

28. *Contact lenses are good for correcting nearsightedness, and so eventually neither contact lenses nor glasses will be needed.* False. Claims have been made that after the use of contact lenses, myopia has stopped progressing. Myopia often stops progressing on its own, however, and no controlled studies have proven that the cases "cured" by the use of contact lenses would not have stopped progressing with no treatment.

29. *Rarely, contact lenses can be lost behind the eye, and even get into the brain.* False. The lens cannot penetrate the conjunctival sac, which lies between it and the back of the eye.

30. *People with only one useful eye need glasses because the eye now does twice the normal work.* False. Either eye is "strong" enough to perform a lifetime of work.

31. *Cheap sunglasses can harm the eyes.* False. See the answers to Nos. 22, 15, and 16. In fact, very little can harm the eyes.

32. *Dark glasses should be worn in bright surroundings (e.g., on the beach or ski slope), since bright sunlight can harm the eyes.* True. Bright sunlight causes the pupil to constrict and cut down the incident light by a sizeable amount. It may cause you to squint, and that may give you a headache. Dark glasses are a comfort measure more than a need in this case. Under bright sunlight, dark adaptation may become temporarily impaired, or ultraviolet keratitis may result.

33. *The color of sunglasses is not important; their color density is.* Essentially true. However, color-deficient patients have even greater difficulty

differentiating colors with a colored lens. These patients should use neutral (gray) lenses.

34. *Polarized sunglasses eliminate the illusory shimmering pools of water often seen on the highway during warm weather.* True. This mirage is a reflection of the sky. On a warm day the air nearest the ground becomes heated and rarified in comparison with that above it and acts as a mirror to reflect the blue sky onto the ground; the viewers then interpret the sky-on-ground as water. Polarized glasses cut out the reflected image.

35. *Ophthalmologist, oculist, and optometrist are all names for eye doctors.* True. An ophthalmologist or oculist (depending upon whether you prefer the Greek or Latin term for eye doctor) is a physician who has specialized in eye diseases and in the testing for spectacles and contact lenses. An optometrist is more akin to a qualified physicist who specializes in the properties of spectacles and contact lenses and their application to different kinds of eyes. The ophthalmologist cannot make a pair of glasses, and the optometrist cannot operate on a cataract. They both can prescribe glasses and contact lenses and this is why people confuse them.

36. *Contact lens wearers have more irritation from their lenses in the summer than during the other seasons.* True. This has to do with the chemistry of air pollution. Exhaust from automobiles contain hydrocarbons. Ultraviolet light converts atmospheric nitrogen into oxides of nitrogen. In a series of photochemical reactions, these compounds combine to form such eye irritants as acrolein, formaldehyde, peroxyacetyl nitrate (PAN), and peroxybenzoyl nitrate (PBzN). In the summertime, the stronger sun produces more of these pollutants. Contact lens wearers are more sensitive than others to air pollutants, and summer is their worst time.

37. *Because outer space is pitch black, good vision is not an important qualification for an astronaut.* It is true that outer space is dark, unless you are in the direct path of the sun. In the space vehicle, however, artificial lighting is used. Under conditions of weightlessness, vision is the only sensory means for orientation in space.

38. *In most states, you need perfect vision in each eye to get a driver's license.* False. Most states require vision correctable to 20/40 in the better or the only eye.

Index